HIV surveillance in the Middle East and North Africa

A handbook for surveillance planners and implementers

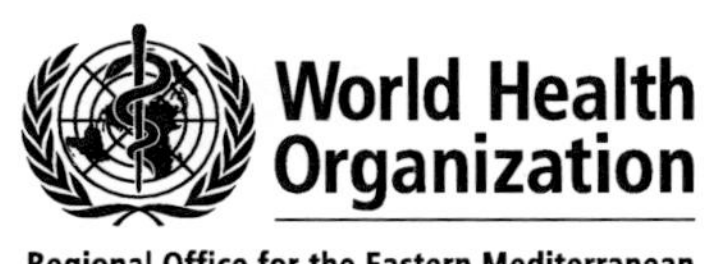

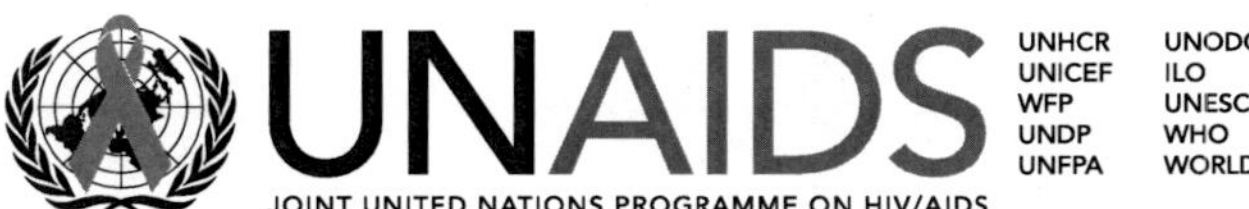

WHO Library Cataloguing in Publication Data

World Health Organization. Regional Office for the Eastern Mediterranean
HIV surveillance in the Middle East and North Africa: a handbook for surveillance planners and implementers / World Health Organization. Regional Office for the Eastern Mediterranean, Joint United Nations Programme on HIV/AIDS
p.
ISBN: 978-92-9021-673-5
ISBN: 978-92-9021-736-7 (online)
1. HIV infections—epidemiology—Middle East—Africa, Northern   2. Health plan implementation   3. Population surveillance—Middle East—Africa, Northern   I. Title   II. Regional Office for the Eastern Mediterranean
III. Joint United Nations Programme on HIV/AIDS
(NLM Classification: WC 503.4)

Contents

Acknowledgements

The World Health Organization Regional Office for the Eastern Mediterranean, the Joint United Nations Programme on HIV/AIDS (UNAIDS) Regional Support Team for the Middle East and North Africa (MENA) and the World Bank have joined their efforts in order to strengthen surveillance of HIV in the Middle East and North Africa.

This handbook is a product of this collaboration. It is meant to accompany those who are involved in HIV surveillance planning and implementation, in particular in countries of the Middle East and North Africa where low-level and concentrated HIV epidemics are predominant. It is designed to provide practical guidance for day-to-day work starting from the design stage of a surveillance system to developing protocols, sampling methodologies and data collections tools for surveillance surveys, the analysis of data and eventually their dissemination and use. It comprises a collection of tools for use in the field.

The handbook was prepared by Ivana Božičević (WHO Collaborating Centre for Capacity Building in HIV/AIDS Surveillance, Croatia), Willi McFarland and H. Fisher Raymond (San Francisco Department of Public Health, USA). Significant contributions were also made by Chris Archibald (Public Health Agency of Canada), Keith Sabin (Centers for Disease Control and Prevention, USA), George Rutherford (University of California San Francisco, USA), Ali-Akhbar Haghdoost (Kerman University of Medical Sciences, Islamic Republic of Iran), Hamidreza Setayesh (UNAIDS), and Jesús M. García Calleja and Gabriele Riedner (WHO).

Introduction

This handbook was developed to assist surveillance officers and programme managers in the planning and implementation of key components of a surveillance system for human immunodeficiency virus (HIV) infection and acquired immunodeficiency syndrome (AIDS) in the Middle East and North Africa where low-level and concentrated HIV epidemics currently predominate; some subregions are also experiencing generalized epidemics.

The US Centers for Disease Control and Prevention (CDC) defines epidemiological surveillance as the "ongoing, systematic collection, analysis, and interpretation of health data" essential to planning, implementation and evaluation of public health practice, closely integrated with the timely dissemination of these data to those who need to know. HIV surveillance is not simply the application of one survey or study method, but rather the design, planning, implementation and use of an integrated system of data collection comprising multiple components.

The framework for the components described in this document is HIV surveillance as outlined by WHO and UNAIDS [1, 2]. Such surveillance emphasizes the need for multiple data sources in order to better understand local HIV epidemics and formulate their appropriate responses. A comprehensive surveillance system must capture the full spectrum of vulnerability and risk factors for HIV transmission as well as key events during the course of HIV infection and related illness until death (see Box 1 and Figure 1).

<table>
<tr><td>

Box 1   Risk and vulnerability

Risk is defined as the probability that a person may become infected with HIV. Unprotected sex, multiple sexual partnerships involving unprotected sex and injection drug use with contaminated injecting equipment are the most important examples of risk behaviour. Risk increases with the prevalence of HIV in the sexual or drug-using network.

Vulnerability to HIV is defined as the extent to which individuals are able to control their risk. Factors that make people vulnerable include: a lack of knowledge about HIV or lack of skills to avoid risk behaviour; inability to obtain condoms, clean needles, or other protection; sex and income inequality that prevents sexual negotiation or contributes to forced sex; and discrimination and stigma, which deter people from changing risk behaviour. These factors, alone or in combination, when shared throughout a community, create collective or community vulnerability. Vulnerability is independent of whether HIV is highly present. Where HIV vulnerability is high it is likely that an individual or community will be less resilient to HIV risk if or when HIV increases within the network.

Adapted from UNAIDS, 2010 [3]

</td></tr>
</table>

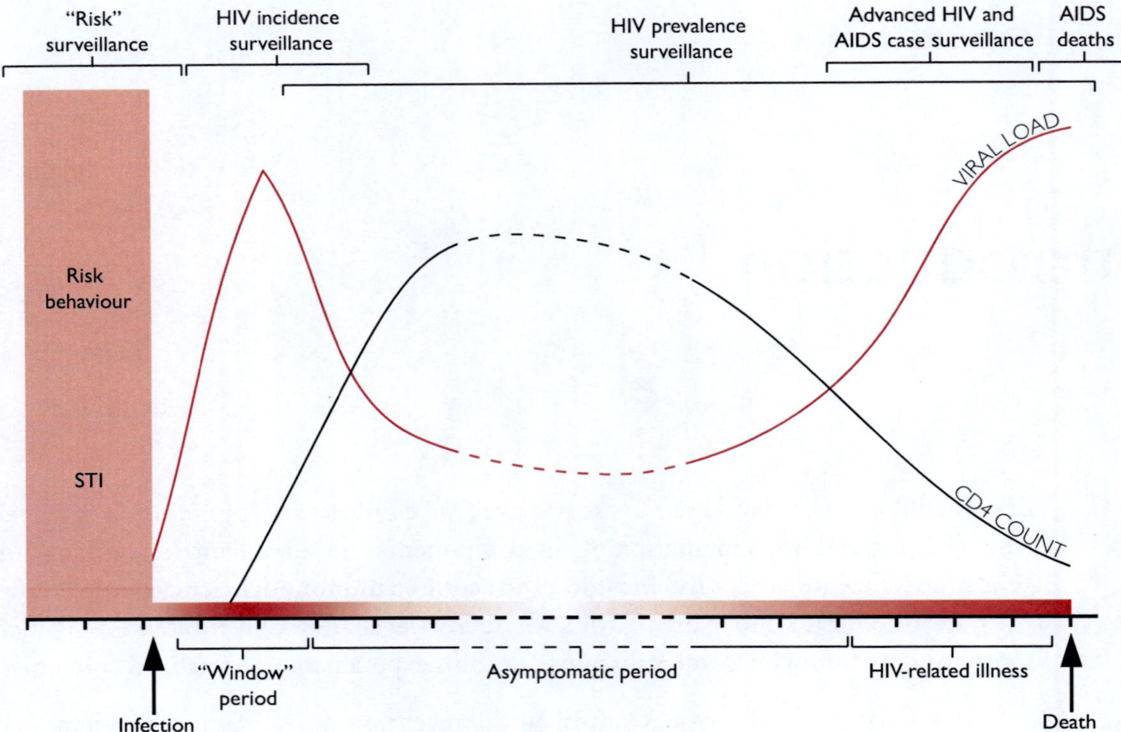

Figure 1   Surveillance of vulnerability, risk and key events during the course of HIV infection and related illness

Key components of a surveillance system include measures of HIV prevalence and incidence in affected populations (e.g. facility-based sentinel surveillance, community prevalence surveys, HIV and AIDS case reporting); measures of prevalence of infections related to HIV (e.g. sexually transmitted infections [STI], tuberculosis [TB] and other opportunistic infections); measures of risk behaviour related to HIV transmission (e.g. unprotected sex, sharing injection equipment, multiple sex partnerships); estimates of the size and make-up of populations at high risk of HIV; measures of the reach and effects of programmes responding to the epidemic; measures of the impact of the responses on morbidity and mortality and the use of other relevant existing information collected for other purposes (e.g. data from voluntary counselling and testing [VCT] programmes, blood bank screening tests, prevention of mother-to-child transmission [PMTCT] programmes, health education outreach and academic research studies).

This publication focuses primarily on the components of surveillance systems that measure and track HIV prevalence and related risk behaviour among most-at-risk populations over time. Specifically, it addresses the design, planning, implementation and use of HIV surveillance data collected through:

- community-based biological and behavioural surveys (i.e. integrated HIV bio-behavioural surveillance or IBBS)
- facility-based HIV prevalence surveys (i.e. sentinel surveillance).

General descriptions of other key components of an HIV surveillance system are also made in this guide with reference to resources for more detail (e.g. HIV and AIDS case reporting, STI surveillance, population size estimation).

Populations of interest in surveillance include the general population, most-at-risk populations, bridging populations and vulnerable populations. Definitions of these populations used in this document are the following.

General population: the general population encompasses all people living in a defined community, e.g. a country, a province or a city. If surveillance data on the general population exclude certain subpopulations, e.g. specific age-groups of the population, foreign workers, refugees or others, this should be stated clearly. The general population is relatively at low risk of HIV exposure in low-level and concentrated HIV epidemics.

Most-at-risk populations include people who use drugs, men who have sex with men, transgendered people and sex workers. Across the world these groups tend to be both vulnerable and at higher risk than others in their locales.

Vulnerable populations are found in all settings. Their risk of acquiring HIV depends on the prevalence of HIV in their networks and their ability to adopt safer behaviour and obtain prevention and treatment commodities and services. For that reason, populations such as people affected by humanitarian emergencies and migration, young people, women, prisoners and people living with disabilities may be at high risk in some places but not in others.

Key populations include both most-at-risk and vulnerable populations, who, while being important to the dynamics of HIV transmission in a setting, are essential partners for an effective response to the epidemic, i.e. they are key to the epidemic and key to the response. Key populations will vary depending on the epidemic and community/country context.

How to use this handbook

This handbook is structured in five parts:

- part 1: introduction and background to surveillance for HIV
- part 2: planning the collection of surveillance information
- part 3: sampling methods for surveillance
- part 4: collecting information from participants in surveillance
- part 5: data management, analysis and interpretation.

Part 1 provides an introduction to HIV surveillance, outlining the broad objectives and components of HIV surveillance systems. It presents examples of successful efforts in establishing and expanding HIV surveillance in the Middle East and North Africa.

Part 2 describes the planning of HIV surveillance, methods and tools for pre-surveillance assessment, the selection of appropriate target groups and staff training needs. Part 2 also introduces methods to estimate the size of populations at high risk of HIV. Related appendixes provide template forms and a protocol outline that can be adapted for local use.

Part 3 provides current methods used for sampling hidden and hard-to-reach populations at risk for HIV. Options are presented for sampling from the community (e.g. cluster sampling, respondent-driven sampling, time-location sampling) and at facilities (i.e. sentinel surveillance). An approach to estimating required sample size is also provided. Related appendixes provide template data collection forms for community- and facility-based surveys.

Part 4 describes biological and behavioural measures used in HIV surveillance and addresses HIV testing principles and algorithms, specimen collection, behavioural data collection and outcome and impact indicators used to evaluate national prevention and care responses. The section also addresses data quality assurance and ethical issues in surveillance systems. Related appendixes contain examples of HIV and AIDS case reporting forms and commercially available HIV assays.

Part 5 outlines the principles of data management, analysis and interpretation of surveillance data for HIV prevention and care planning. Guidelines are provided for the evaluation of surveillance systems emphasizing planning for surveillance as a continuous activity.

A comprehensive HIV surveillance system has to be standardized and consistent over time, yet also flexible, timely and sensitive to new conditions affecting the epidemic and new technologies for collecting and managing information. While the primary focus of these guidelines is on basic HIV prevalence and risk behaviour data for surveillance, we recommend incremental improvements in components. High priority rests with the establishment of basic needs of surveillance systems for the Middle East and North African context. We provide overviews and references to other activities to be integrated into future, more advanced surveillance systems or on a pilot basis for some more developed locations. Looking ahead, future components may include:

- incident, recent and acute HIV infection surveillance
- surveillance for diseases transmitted in similar ways to HIV (e.g. other STI, hepatitis C [HCV])
- HIV and AIDS case reporting
- HIV morbidity surveillance (e.g. CD4 T-lymphocyte, viral load, primary and secondary opportunistic infections, AIDS-related cancers and other associated conditions)
- surveillance for care and treatment of people living with HIV (e.g. use of prophylaxis, antiretroviral therapy [ART], prevention of mother-to-child transmission treatments)
- surveillance for primary and in-care antiretroviral drug resistance and early warning indicator surveillance
- AIDS mortality surveillance
- programmatic, research and ancillary data for use in surveillance.

Strengthening the basic components of HIV surveillance for the Middle East and North Africa will help capitalize on the still-existing opportunity to halt the wider spread of HIV to persons at risk, their immediate contacts and the wider population. Components of surveillance systems that are well developed in one part of the region or country may act models for further strengthening surveillance elsewhere. The diversity of HIV epidemics across the countries in the region and the country-specific organization of health care systems will undoubtedly reflect diverse HIV surveillance systems, tailored according to local needs and yet based on the common principles of surveillance presented in this document.

References

1   *Initiating second generation HIV surveillance systems: practical guidelines.* UNAIDS/WHO Working Group on Global HIV/AIDS/STI Surveillance. Geneva, UNAIDS/WHO, 2002.

2   *Guidelines for second generation HIV surveillance: the next decade.* UNAIDS/WHO Working Group on Global HIV/AIDS and STI Surveillance. Geneva, UNAIDS/WHO, 2000.

3   *What's preventing prevention: campaign policy briefing 1.* International HIV/AIDS Alliance, 2010. Available at http://www.aidsalliance.org/includes/Document/ Prevention%20campaign/Campaign-Policy-Briefing-1.pdf.

Part I

Introduction and background to surveillance for HIV

1.1

Overview of HIV surveillance

1.1.1 Definition and objectives of HIV surveillance

Epidemiological surveillance is defined as the ongoing systematic collection, recording, analysis, interpretation and dissemination of data reflecting the current health status of a community or population. It is essential to planning, implementation and evaluation of public health practice and is closely integrated with the timely dissemination of these data to those who need to know. The definition emphasizes the use of data for public health action, not simply the collection of information as an end in itself.

The objectives of HIV surveillance include the provision of timely and reliable information for:

- advocacy for resources for prevention and care, mobilization of political commitment
- appropriate resource allocation between affected populations and areas
- effective targeting of prevention, care and support programmes
- monitoring and evaluation of the aggregate impact of programmes
- developing new programmes
- informing the public
- tracking the leading edge of the epidemic
- projecting future care and prevention needs
- identifying information gaps and guiding research to fill those gaps
- making health policies to maximize the effectiveness of the above.

With respect to HIV, a surveillance system enables evidence-based public health decision-making for HIV care, prevention and control. HIV surveillance activities need to be integrated into a comprehensive system that captures the full spectrum of HIV and AIDS with measures to identify the populations at most risk, the direction of the spread of infection, the factors driving transmission and the impact of efforts to prevent, treat and mitigate the individual and societal impact of infection.

HIV has features that distinguish it from many other infections, including multiple modes of transmission (e.g. through sex, by sharing injection equipment, through blood transfusion, during pregnancy, at delivery and through breast milk), lifelong infection, little evidence of immunity, a long period between infection and the manifestation of disease and associations with illegal and highly stigmatized behaviour. There is no vaccine nor is there a cure. Its treatment is costly and of life-long duration. Its prevention has proven difficult. In recent years, HIV has been singled out for special international funding and therefore maintains a high political profile. These properties of HIV necessitate several considerations when in designing surveillance systems, in particular:

- HIV infections enter different geographic areas and populations at different times and spread at different rates and by different modes[1]
- HIV infections are not uniformly distributed in a population
- many groups most vulnerable to infection are also subject to prejudice, discrimination and legal proscription
- extreme care in maintaining confidentiality is required given the potential legal and social harm that may befall persons when it becomes known they are living with HIV
- HIV is associated with many other acute and chronic infections and diseases
- a wide range of data sources, methods, measures and activities are required for HIV surveillance.

1.1.2   Basic measures of comprehensive HIV surveillance

In order to meet the above goals and objectives, HIV surveillance data centre on several basic epidemiological, behavioural, social and programmatic measures. These measures include:

- the prevalence of and temporal trends in HIV infection (when HIV prevalence is low or difficult to measure, other infectious diseases that share modes of transmission with HIV are often used as proxies; for example, other STI [e.g. syphilis, herpes simplex virus 2 (HSV-2), gonorrhoea, chlamydia] and other bloodborne pathogens such as HCV)
- the incidence of HIV, although difficult to measure in most settings
- the prevalence and incidence of opportunistic infections
- the prevalence of and temporal trends in sexual risk behaviour that increase risk of HIV acquisition and transmission (e.g. unprotected vaginal sex with a non-cohabiting partner, unprotected anal sex between men of different HIV serostatus)
- the prevalence of and temporal trends in drug-use behaviour directly and indirectly related to HIV acquisition and transmission (e.g. the sharing of injection drug use equipment, consumption of alcohol or other drugs that affect condom use)
- the correlates of HIV infection, other related infections and risk behaviour to identify populations at highest risk, specific factors driving transmission and protective factors slowing the spread of infection

---

[1]   The transmission dynamics of HIV within populations are determined by complex interactions involving the behavioural characteristics of individuals, the background prevalence of infection, other biological parameters (for example, prevalence of STI, circumcision status) and the availability and accessibility of health care. Interpretation of HIV epidemics should be done by carefully examining the complex interplay of these and other factors. The most immediate determinants of HIV and STI spread in any population are the three components of the rate of spread model described by Anderson and May [15]: transmission efficiency per contact (infectivity), rate of contact between infected and susceptible individuals and the duration of infectiousness. These components are influenced by other factors. For example, infectivity is determined by factors such as condom use, presence of other STI and circumcision status. Duration of infectiousness depends on the pathogen characteristics, but also on the provision of health care services (screening and treatment). Transmission efficiency (the probability of HIV transmission) differs according to the route of transmission, but also according to other parameters such as viral load (the amount of virus in body fluids) and presence of STI. The risk of HIV transmission is higher in the presence of high viral load in an infected person, which occurs in the early and late stages of disease. Higher viral load in the blood corresponds to higher viral load in genital fluids (semen and vaginal secretions), and effective treatment with antiretroviral therapy (drugs used to fight HIV infection) lowers the viral load in blood and perhaps also in genital fluids. The efficiency of HIV transmission varies according to the route of transmission and according to the viral load, exposure to antiretroviral therapy and presence of other cofactors such as STI. Various studies have estimated HIV transmission as follows (likelihood of transmission per exposure): blood transfusion: 90%–100%; mother-to-child transmission: 15%–20%, with breastfeeding 35%–40%; vaginal intercourse: 0.03%–0.2%; anal intercourse: 0.06%–3.0%; intravenous drug injection: 0.24%–0.65%.

- measures of access, reach, intensity and use of HIV care, prevention and control programmes
- patterns of health-seeking behaviour and the types of providers and services being sought
- self-perception of risk, basic knowledge, beliefs and attitudes towards HIV and people living with HIV
- linkages between populations at high risk of HIV to each other and to populations at lower risk (e.g. the proportion of sex workers who inject drugs or have sex partners who inject drugs, the proportion of men who have sex with men who are also married or have other female partners)
- AIDS deaths.

Because **HIV prevalence** and **HIV incidence** are central measures for surveillance, clarification of their definitions and distinctions is warranted.

- **Prevalence** is the proportion of HIV-infected persons in a specific group. It is a direct measure of the burden of disease in a population. Prevalence is usually expressed as point prevalence, which refers to prevalence at a single point in time. When specifically determined by testing serum for HIV antibody, it is often referred to as seroprevalence.
- **Incidence** is the rate of new HIV infections occurring in a group during a specific period of time. Incidence measures the rate of increase or decrease of the epidemic.

Prevalence of HIV infection in younger age groups, such as those between 15 and 19 years old or 15 and 24 years old, is considered to be a proxy for HIV incidence because their period of sexual activity is relatively short and more recent. For example, in antenatal clinic (ANC) sentinel surveillance HIV prevalence in women aged 15–24 years old serves as a proxy for HIV incidence in the general population (or for the population of young people).

In addition to the specific measures, HIV surveillance seeks an understanding of the context and conditions that may foster the spread of HIV and the resources that can be brought to bear in the response to the epidemic. Such information may originate from surveillance activities directly (e.g. formative assessments of most-at-risk populations) or from other sources (e.g. prevention and care policies and strategic plans). Moreover, surveillance data also require information on the "denominator" for the populations at risk. For example, HIV prevalence in most-at-risk populations require an estimate of the size of the population (e.g. the number of men having sex with men [MSM], female sex workers [FSW] or injection drug users [IDU] in an area) in order to make appropriate resource allocation decisions.

Local, national and international bodies specifically define measures or "indicators" used to compare populations, geographic areas and programme impact over time. Examples of internationally adopted indicators are those defined by UNGASS [United Nations General Assembly Special Session on HIV/AIDS, Guidelines on Construction of Core Indicators: 2010 Reporting, UNAIDS/09.10E/JC1676E, Geneva, March 2009], with many originating from HIV surveillance data such as:

- Core Indicator 7: percentage of women and men aged 15–49 who received HIV testing in the previous 12 months and who know their results

- Core Indicator 9: percentage of most-at-risk populations reached by HIV prevention programmes
- Core Indicator 15: percentage of young women and men who have had sexual intercourse before the age of 15
- Core Indicator 18: percentage of female and male sex workers reporting use of a condom with their most recent client
- Core Indicator 21: percentage of injection drug users who reported using sterile injection equipment the most recent time they injected
- Core Indicator 22: percentage of young women and men aged 15 to 24 who are HIV-infected
- Core Indicator 23: percentage of most-at-risk populations who are HIV-infected.

1.1.3 Components of a comprehensive HIV surveillance system

A comprehensive HIV surveillance system encompasses the full spectrum of HIV and AIDS. This includes not only the period from HIV infection until death due to AIDS-related morbidities, but also the behaviour that leads to infection, the risk factors for transmission and social and economic conditions that foster the spread of HIV as well as the impact of HIV on families, populations and society.

One principle of surveillance is that the mix of surveillance activities is flexible and adapted to the appropriate stage of the epidemic. According to the WHO/UNAIDS classification, there are three stages of HIV epidemic: low-level, concentrated and generalized [3]. Box 1.1 below describes the classification system according to HIV prevalence. Low-level epidemics are defined by an HIV prevalence that does not exceed 5% in any defined subpopulation and is less than 1% in the general population (as measured in pregnant women as a proxy). In concentrated epidemics, HIV prevalence is over 5% in at least one subpopulation and less than 1% in pregnant women. In generalized epidemics, HIV is firmly established in the general population and exceeds 1% among pregnant women.

Figure 1.1 below illustrates key components of surveillance in **low-level epidemics**. Population-based surveys, such as demographic and health surveys (DHS) provide needed data on the general level of HIV knowledge and some types of risk behaviour in the general population. However, in low-level epidemics household surveys will not detect sufficient

---

Box 1.1 WHO and UNAIDS classification of HIV/AIDS epidemics

Low-level	HIV prevalence has not consistently exceeded 5% in any defined subpopulation and is <1% in pregnant women
Concentrated	HIV prevalence is consistently >5% in at least one defined subpopulation and is <1% in pregnant women
Generalized	HIV prevalence is firmly established in the general population and is consistently >1% in pregnant women

numbers of infections for precise inference of the magnitude of infection or direction of spread of HIV. HIV testing in DHS-like surveys is therefore not recommended in countries or regions with low-level epidemics. Rather, they serve to provide measures of the general knowledge of HIV in the area, levels of risk behaviour in the general population and potential bridges to high-risk populations. The costs of population-based household surveys prohibit repeating them more frequently than once every four to five years.

Household surveys are also unlikely to detect sufficient numbers of most-at-risk population members. Persons participating in household surveys are likely to deny the stigmatized behaviour that often define most-at-risk populations, such as male–male sex, exchanging sex for money or illicit drug use. Therefore, rapid qualitative assessments of most-at-risk populations are conducted in the locations where they visibly congregate. These types of activities, which can lead to more systematic surveillance surveys, include PLACE (priorities for locating AIDS control and evaluation) or RARE (rapid assessment, response and evaluation) where the goal is to quickly gain information on the populations at highest risk, the places where risk occurs and to deliver an appropriate prevention response. Guidelines on how to conduct PLACE can be found at http://www.cpc.unc.edu/ measure/leadership/place.html. Additional information on RARE methods can be found at http://www.who.int/docstore/HIV/Core/Index.html

These qualitative efforts can form a foundation for more systematic data collection on most-at-risk populations. As described elsewhere in these guidelines, mapping of the venues where most-at-risk populations concentrate provides a sampling frame for probability-based surveys to obtain representative estimates of HIV prevalence and risk behaviour. Such surveys can also produce most-at-risk population size estimates when combined with other procedures such as capture-recapture and multiplier methods. A brief introduction to most-at-risk population size estimation methods is included in this guide. For further information, see: *Guidelines for estimating the size of populations most at risk to HIV*. Geneva, UNAIDS/WHO, 2010; and *Estimating the size of populations at risk for HIV*. Arlington, Virginia, Family Health International, 2003.

In low-level epidemics, HIV testing in antenatal clinics (ANC) for the purpose of surveillance (i.e. sentinel surveillance) is also unlikely to detect sufficient numbers of infections for statistical inference and is therefore not advised or limited to a few sites in large urban areas. Moreover, sentinel surveillance is typically conducted by delinking

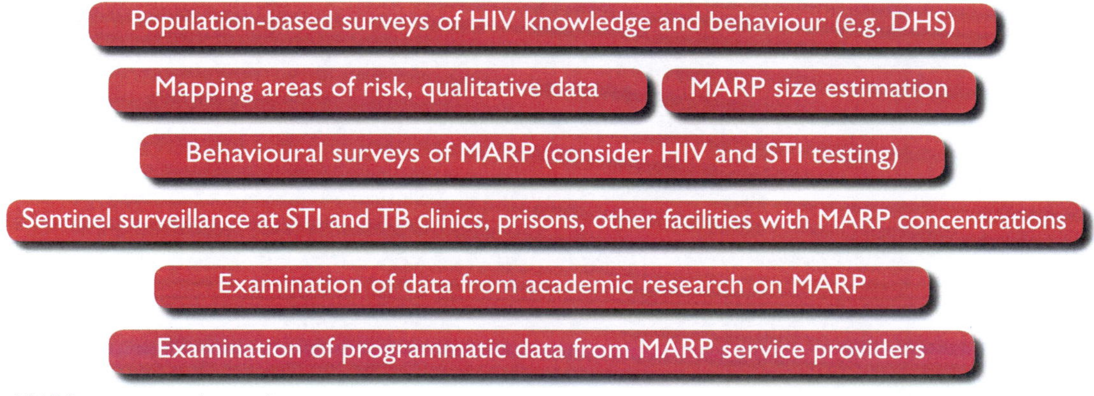

MARP: most-at-risk population.

Figure I.I Low-level epidemics: key surveillance components

serological results from individuals and does not collect risk behaviour data. However, other facilities that include large numbers of most-at-risk populations may be among the first places to detect the appearance of HIV in a country or region and provide inference on the prevalence of HIV in most-at-risk populations. For example, HIV infection may reach substantial levels at STI clinics, TB clinics, drug detoxification or rehabilitation centres, prisons and employment sites for occupations where sex worker contact is often high (e.g. long-distance lorry drivers, military and other uniformed personnel, seafarers) even in low-level epidemic areas by virtue of having a high proportion of most-at-risk populations present. The basic principles and methods of sentinel surveillance are covered in this guide. For further details, see *Guidelines for conducting HIV sentinel serosurveys among pregnant women and other groups*. Geneva, UNAIDS/WHO, 2003. UNAIDS/03.49E, available at http://data.unaids.org/Publications/IRC-pub06/JC954-anc-Serosurveys_Guidelines_en.pdf. Additional guidance on HIV surveillance among TB patients can be found in *Guidelines for HIV surveillance among tuberculosis patients*. Geneva, UNAIDS/WHO, 2004. UNAIDS/04.30E, available at http://data.unaids.org/Publications/IRC-pub06/JC740-hiv-tb_surveillance_en.pdf.

In addition to sentinel surveillance in facilities with high concentrations of most-at-risk populations, careful examination of academic research of most-at-risk populations and routine data collected by programmes serving most-at-risk populations should form a key component of surveillance in low-level epidemics.

Concentrated epidemics (Figure 1.2) require many of the same surveillance components as low-level epidemics, such as periodic population-based surveys of HIV-related knowledge and behaviour (DHS), examination of research study data and analysis of routine programmatic data on most-at-risk populations. In contrast to low-level epidemics, concentrated epidemics require expansion of HIV testing as the higher prevalence increases the likelihood of detecting sufficient numbers of infections for meaningful interpretation. Population-based surveys, such as DHS or AIDS indicator surveys (AIS), may consider HIV testing; however, HIV prevalence will remain very low, and

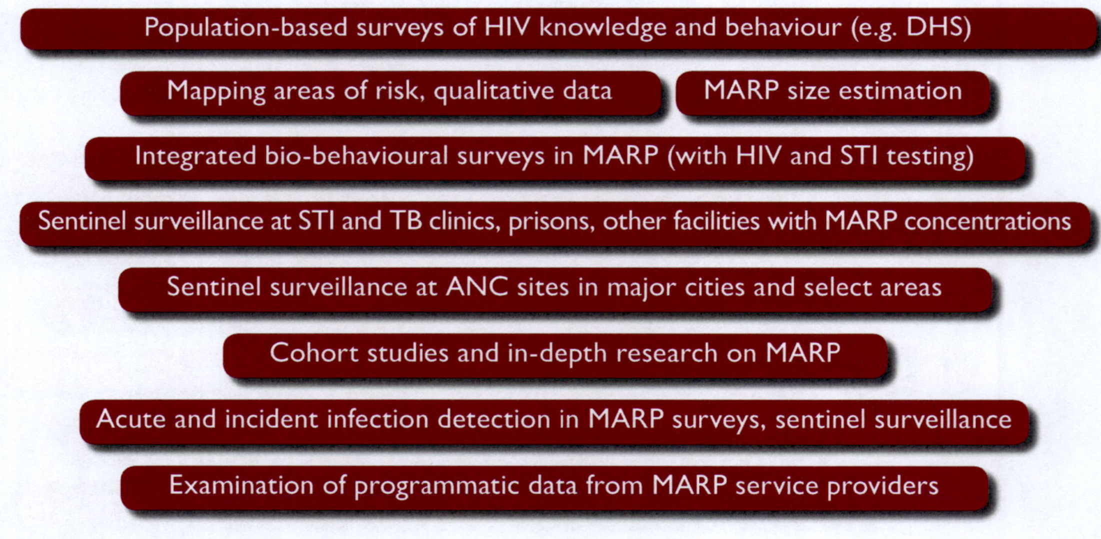

MARP: most-at-risk population.

Figure 1.2 Concentrated epidemics key surveillance components

denial of stigmatized behaviour in household surveys may obscure the true risk factors for infection. Instead, the key surveillance component for measuring HIV prevalence in most-at-risk populations is referred to as an integrated bio-behavioural survey (IBBS). IBBS is conducted with verification of most-at-risk population membership and, unlike sentinel surveillance, links HIV serological results to the reported risk behaviour. Given the central role that most-at-risk populations play in the low-level and concentrated epidemics found in the Middle East and North Africa, the methods and options for IBBS are the major focus of this guide.

Sentinel surveillance at facilities with high numbers of most-at-risk populations remains a key component of HIV surveillance in concentrated epidemics. In addition, sentinel surveillance among women attending ANC is warranted in a few locations, such as large urban centres where HIV usually appears first or in specific locations where HIV prevalence among most-at-risk populations is high (e.g. port cities, towns on lorry routes, border towns).

However, in concentrated epidemics widespread coverage of ANC sentinel surveillance is not advised as most locations (e.g. rural areas) will remain at very low HIV prevalence as long as most infections are concentrated in most-at-risk populations.

In addition to conventional HIV antibody testing to measure prevalence of infection, assays to detect acute and recent infection in specific studies of most-at-risk populations may be feasible in concentrated epidemics. For example, the BED assay (see section 4.3.3) may be applied to research studies of most-at-risk populations or facility-based sentinel surveillance specimens. The specific requirements for HIV incidence surveillance are beyond the scope of this guide and remain under development at present.

In **generalized epidemics** (Figure 1.3), HIV infection has become firmly established in the general population. HIV testing within general population-based surveys (e.g. DHS and AIS) detects sufficient numbers of HIV infection for surveillance goals. Because such surveys are costly and only done every four to five years, HIV prevalence trends in the general population are tracked through ANC sentinel surveillance using pregnant women as a proxy with extensive national coverage, in urban and rural areas, on an annual or

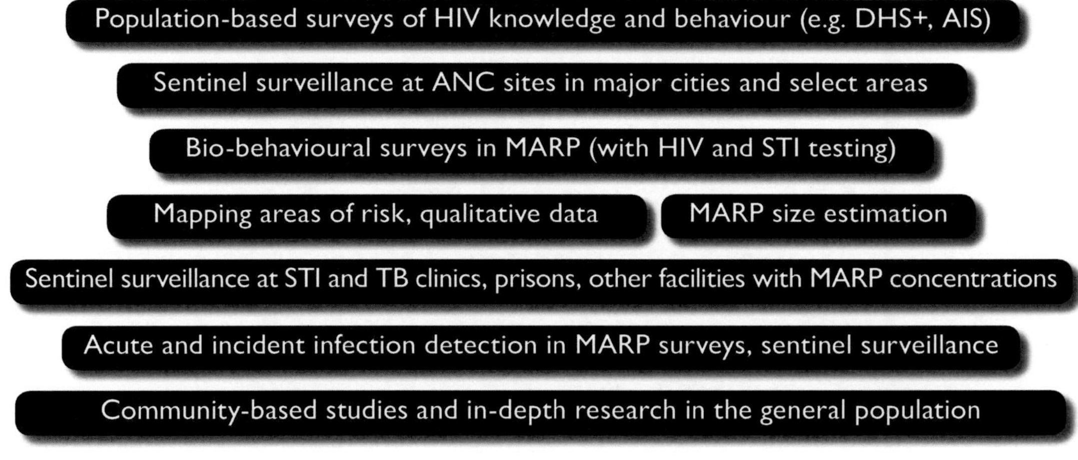

MARP: most-at-risk population.

Figure 1.3 Generalized epidemics key surveillance components

biennial basis. DHS+ (i.e. DHS with HIV testing) data are used to "calibrate" HIV prevalence at ANC sites by making side-by-side comparisons.

Although subpopulations at high risk may continue to contribute disproportionately to the spread of HIV, sexual networking, risk behaviour and the background prevalence of infection in the general population are sufficient to sustain an epidemic independent of subpopulations at higher risk of infection. Nonetheless, HIV prevalence and behavioural measures among most-at-risk populations are increasingly recognized as key components of surveillance even within generalized epidemics.

Analysis of data from academic research on the general population and most-at-risk populations and routine examination of programmatic data for services to the general population continue to be ongoing activities in generalized epidemics to complement other components of surveillance.

Several components are integral parts of a comprehensive surveillance system in **all epidemic stages** (Figure 1.4).

In virtually all countries of the world, there are legal mandates and systems in place to report the occurrence of selected infectious diseases and health conditions of particular high priority by virtue of morbidity and mortality. HIV and/or AIDS cases diagnosed are usually required by law to be reported—in principle. For many areas of the world, severe underreporting occurs due to lack of diagnostic capability (e.g. HIV testing, CD4 testing, definitive diagnoses for opportunistic infections [OI]), lack of knowledge of reporting

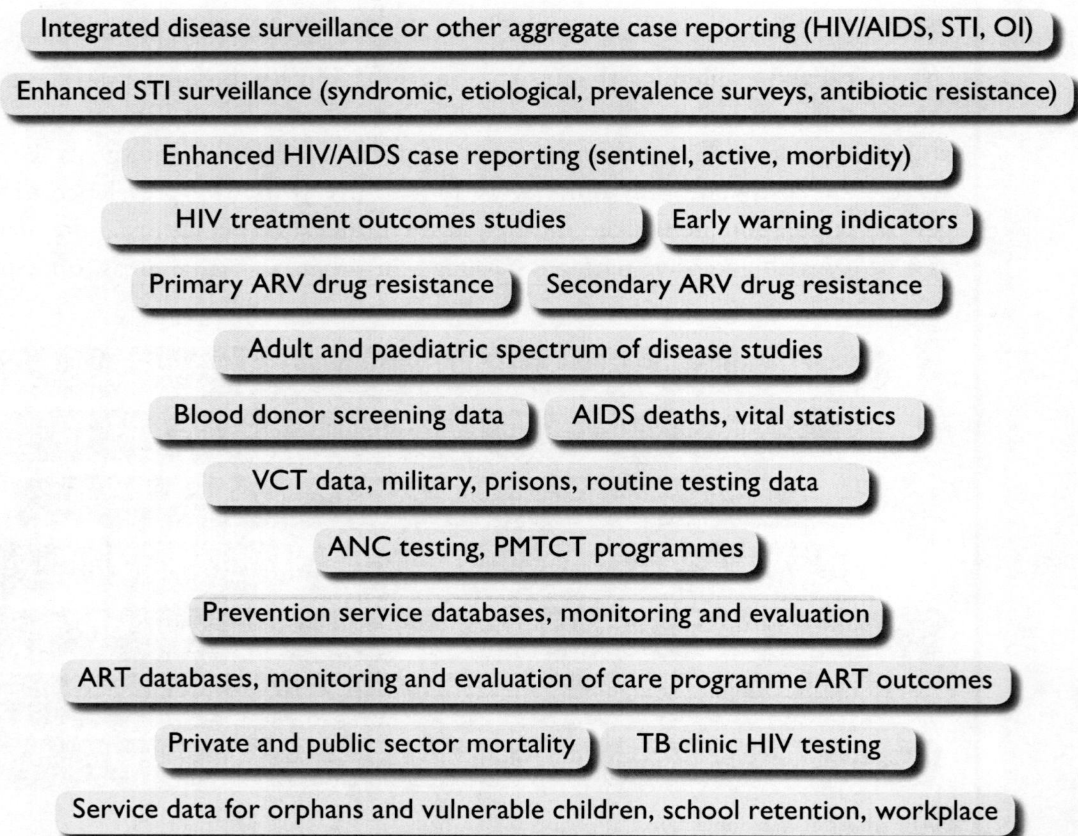

Figure 1.4 Surveillance components for all epidemic stages

requirements by care providers and limited resources. In addition, systems that do not adequately filter out duplicate reported cases may overestimate diagnoses from some facilities. Nonetheless, reporting diagnosed cases of HIV and AIDS is a core surveillance activity in all stages of the epidemic, and such systems need to be strengthened in the Middle East and North Africa. However, HIV and AIDS case reporting is beyond the scope of this present guide.

Some regions employ an "integrated disease surveillance" (IDS) approach to case reporting, whereby cases are aggregated by pathogen at the facility, district, province and national levels (e.g. monthly counts). Other areas may conduct "sentinel case reporting" in which a few selected, large facilities record individual diagnoses. In the particular case of STI, some areas conduct enhanced surveillance components which include reporting syndromic (e.g. genital ulcer, urethral discharge) or etiological (e.g. syphilis, gonorrhoea, chlamydia) diagnoses, syndromic validation studies, prevalence surveys and antibiotic resistance studies.

With the scale-up of antiretroviral therapy (ART) internationally, HIV surveillance has been expanded to include outcomes related to HIV care. Although not included in the current guide, advanced surveillance activities include studies of HIV treatment outcomes (e.g. morbidity and mortality, discontinuation, co-infections, co-morbidities), primary and secondary antiretroviral medicine resistance surveillance beginning with early warning indicators, longitudinal studies on the adult and paediatric spectrums of disease, and enhanced AIDS mortality surveillance (e.g. strengthening national vital statistics, private and public sector employee mortality).

The careful examination of routine or programmatic data is also a part of a comprehensive surveillance system in all stages of the epidemic. These include HIV testing in select populations, such as blood donors or military personnel, provider-initiated HIV testing for prevention of mother-to-child transmission (PMTCT), TB clinic HIV testing and general voluntary counselling and testing (VCT) data. However, these data should not be considered as representative samples of the entire population at risk as they include persons seeking and accessing services or are highly selected groups. Other sources of information may also enhance the interpretation of surveillance data. Data routinely collected by prevention and care service providers in the context of monitoring and evaluation provide context for the interpretation of other HIV surveillance data and for the formulation of appropriate responses to the epidemic. Academic research data can provide more depth than sentinel surveillance or IBBS surveys, particularly qualitative research of high-quality and longitudinal cohort data.

1.1.4 Overview of HIV sentinel surveillance and integrated bio-behavioural surveys

The focus of this guide is on the planning and implementation of two central components of surveillance: clinic- or facility-based HIV sentinel surveillance and community-based bio-behavioural surveys. This section provides an overview of the methods of these surveillance components; greater detail is provided in subsequent chapters.

As introduced above, **sentinel surveillance** is conducted in facilities, clinics or sites that capture or serve populations at highest risk for HIV infection. They approximate cross-sectional samples of the particular populations included in the facility. In low-level and concentrated epidemics, these facilities include STI, TB and drug dependence treatment centres or prisons, workplaces or other institutional settings where most-at-risk populations are concentrated and where HIV infection may appear first in a population. In generalized epidemics, sentinel sites are typically ANC, using HIV prevalence among pregnant women as a proxy for the general population.

Sentinel surveillance focuses on monitoring trends in HIV prevalence. Some sociodemographic data may be collected, but behavioural data are limited to what is routinely collected by the site for purposes other than surveillance. For example, the typical approach is that HIV testing is by **unlinked anonymous testing** (UAT), conducted on blood collected for other purposes (e.g. syphilis testing). In this approach, only data routinely collected are abstracted (e.g. sociodemographic data) and no specific HIV-related questions are asked. The design has the advantages of consistency over time and limiting participation bias, but data on the risk factors and behaviour driving the HIV epidemic are usually not included. Moreover, most-at-risk population membership is only implied and not verified.

Community-based **integrated bio-behavioural surveillance** (IBBS) surveys are conducted as cross-sectional surveys while linking HIV test results to the reported behaviour of participants. In this manner, most-at-risk population membership is verified, and risk factors and behaviour are directly linked to HIV infection. Because most-at-risk populations are typically stigmatized and engage in illegal behaviour, they are typically hidden and hard to reach, and obtaining representative samples is challenging. At present, a few sampling options are in common use worldwide and are described in detail in this guide. These include the following.

Cluster-based sampling is based on the random selection of fixed places where the target population can be found and enumerated with relative confidence. A random, consecutive (all persons in sequence) or systematic (every nth person) sample is then drawn at the location gauging the number to be proportional to the population size (or adjusted in analysis to be representative). For groups in the general population or in specific occupations, these may include clusters of houses or residences, schools, workplaces, military barracks or prisons. For FSW, these may include brothels, entertainment centres or other places where direct or indirect FSW are employed. For IDU, these may include prisons, rehabilitation centres or drug dependence treatment centres. Few such eligible places exist for MSM. The principle behind cluster sampling is that the target population can be efficiently reached in visible sites and can be enrolled into the IBBS in approximate proportion to their relative sizes at the sites.

In many areas, most-at-risk populations congregate in particular locations, but their exact numbers are not known or mobility through the sites is very high. In such situations, **time-location sampling** (TLS) can be used to approximate cluster-based sampling. In TLS, a roster of all locations where the most-at-risk populations can be found is made along with the days of the week and times of highest activity, called **venue-day-time** (VDT) **clusters**. A sample of VDT is randomly selected and persons at the VDT are randomly, consecutively or systematically recruited. The representativeness of the sample is based on the enumeration of the most-at-risk populations at the venue from formative assessment or at the time of recruitment.

When the most-at-risk population does not congregate in certain areas/venues or is truly hidden, then **respondent-driven sampling** (RDS) can provide a diverse and potentially representative sample. RDS is a long chain-referral process similar to snowball sampling in which members of the most-at-risk population recruit peers from their social networks. The number of referrals is limited to ensure recruitment chains penetrate diverse social circles. Biases in recruitment patterns are corrected for by statistically adjusting estimates for network sizes and the tendencies of persons to recruit others like themselves.

Of note, careful formative assessment, potentially beginning with a PLACE or RARE study, is required for the above IBBS survey methods. Details of this formative phase are provided in subsequent chapters of this guide.

1.1.5 HIV surveillance in the Middle East and North Africa

For the purposes of this guide, the Middle East and North Africa comprises Member States of the WHO Eastern Mediterranean Region and countries covered by the UNAIDS Middle East and North Africa Region. These are: Afghanistan, Algeria, Bahrain, Djibouti, Egypt, Islamic Republic of Iran, Iraq, Jordan, Kuwait, Lebanon, Libyan Arab Jamahiriya, Morocco, Oman, Pakistan, Qatar, Saudi Arabia, Somalia, Sudan, Syrian Arab Republic, Tunisia, United Arab Emirates, Yemen and the occupied Palestinian territory.

There are many driving factors for HIV transmission in the Middle East and North Africa. Where available, data suggest high prevalence of risky behaviour among injection drug users, overlap between drug use and sex work and gaps in coverage with harm reduction interventions. Other potentially facilitating factors for the increased risk of HIV spread include consequences of conflicts with increased vulnerability and high numbers of refugees and internally displaced persons (Afghanistan, Iraq, occupied Palestinian territory, Somalia and Sudan), large numbers of migrant workers from and outside the region, marginalization of most-at-risk populations and insufficient scale of the prevention programmes [9, 10].

The region is diverse with respect to the levels of HIV epidemics. The southern part of Sudan, Djibouti and some parts of Somalia face generalized epidemics where HIV prevalence is consistently above 1% in pregnant women in wide areas of the country [11, 12]. Afghanistan, Islamic Republic of Iran, Libyan Arab Jamahiriya, Oman and Pakistan have concentrated epidemics largely among IDU. Recent data from some countries including Egypt, Sudan and Tunisia suggest an elevated HIV prevalence among MSM [14]. Most countries of the region are considered to be in the low-level epidemic stage though more reliable data on HIV prevalence in groups most-at-risk are needed to estimate the levels of HIV epidemics with greater certainty.

Surveys assessing HIV-related knowledge, attitudes and behaviour in different countries of the region suggest that young people are not sufficiently aware of HIV and lack adequate knowledge of modes of HIV transmission and prevention.

Well developed HIV surveillance systems are lacking in most of the countries of the region. This limits considerably the understanding of the size and characteristics of the HIV epidemic in the region as well as the opportunities for evidence-based HIV intervention. The current estimates noted above are based on available data, but improved data are needed to more effectively monitor the epidemic and to guide programmes and policies.

In most countries, HIV surveillance consists mainly of HIV and AIDS case reporting, which is unable to provide estimates of the burden of infection as it relies on reporting practices of physicians and the patterns of HIV testing. Nevertheless, there are numerous good examples of successful efforts to improve surveillance. Such examples include HIV serosurveillance in ANC, TB and STI clinic patients in Sudan and Somalia. The Islamic Republic of Iran has HIV serosurveillance surveys in prisons. Annual rounds of bio-behavioural surveillance surveys among most-at-risk populations have been conducted in a number of sites in Pakistan (among male and female sex workers, *hijra*[1], IDU and lorry drivers). Annual sentinel facility-based surveillance among sex workers is carried out in Morocco. In recent years bio-behavioural surveys among most-at-risk populations have been carried out by an increasing number of countries including Afghanistan, Islamic Republic of Iran, Pakistan, Lebanon, Egypt, Tunisia, Morocco, Sudan, Somalia and Yemen.

---

[1] In south Asia, *hijra* are members of a community of male transvestites or eunuchs, traditionally performing as singers or dancers at religious festivals or at social occasions such as weddings. Sometimes they get involved in sex work and are in such situations a target group for surveillance.

1.2

Examples of successful HIV surveillance efforts in the Middle East and North Africa

This section provides examples of HIV surveillance activities in Somalia and Pakistan established as the first rounds of clinic-based and community-based surveillance surveys in those countries, respectively. We share lessons learned and challenges encountered while conducting surveillance and during data interpretation to help build better quality surveillance systems in the future. Details of the methods used are described in subsequent chapters of this guide.

1.2.1 Example of clinic-based HIV surveillance surveys in Somalia

Comprehensive HIV sentinel serosurveillance in Somalia was initiated in 2004, though a smaller-scale HIV seroprevalence survey was conducted in 1999 in the Somaliland region. The aims of the HIV and STI prevalence surveys conducted in 2004 were to generate baseline HIV and STI data for Somalia; to determine the current prevalence of HIV and STI infections in ANC, STI and TB patients; and to provide information for advocacy, planning and monitoring of interventions.

Methods

Sites for surveillance were selected in four regions in the north-west zone of Somalia, three regions in the north-east, and five in the central/south zone. The criteria used for selecting the regions included the population density in urban areas and the security situation. The criteria used for selecting the sites in the regions were accessibility, availability of staff, adequate number of attendees and feasibility of implementing future interventions. The overall number of sites where prevalence surveys were conducted was 22. The sample size was set at 350 per ANC site, assuming an HIV prevalence of 2% (with the estimated 95% CI = 0.5–3.5). The sample size for TB and STI patients was set at 250 per site, assuming a prevalence of 5% (with the estimated 95% CI = 2.3–7.7). The sample size for the STI prevalence study in symptomatic patients was set at 250 (95% CI = 2.3–7.7), and for asymptomatic patients 500 (95% CI = 3.1–6.9). Patients were included by consecutive sampling until the sample size was reached. The data collection period lasted

12–16 weeks. The inclusion criteria were: resident in one of the three zones of Somalia[1] for at least one year; and age group 15–49 years for ANC and STI patients and 15–59 years for TB patients.

Training workshops were organized for all sites, and topics included site selection, recruitment of patients, administration of data collection forms, blood sample collection, coding, storage, transportation, laboratory testing, confidentiality, ethical issues, quality assurance, supervision and survey management strategies. Supervisory visits were carried out during data collection.

Data collection forms were completed by nurses abstracting clinic data. The specimen containers were labelled using codes that consisted of the patient number, town code, facility code and date. On-site testing was done for syphilis by rapid plasma regain test (RPR) and for HIV (by Capillus HIV1/HIV2). After this initial testing on sites, samples were transported to the reference laboratories in the zones. All samples were retested using Capillus HIV1/HIV2 and Determine (both rapid tests for HIV) and RPR and *Treponema pallidum* haemagglutination assay (TPHA). Syphilis and haemoglobin results were provided to patients, while separate aliquots were coded following unlinked anonymous testing (UAT) procedures. All positive and all negative samples were stored at –70 °C and transported to the WHO collaborative centre for external quality control at the University of Nairobi. Urine and vaginal swabs were collected from ANC attendees and cervical and urethral swabs from STI patients and stored at –70 °C for onward transportation to the University of Nairobi to be tested for gonorrhoea and chlamydia using polymerase chain reaction (PCR). All women from whom blood was drawn for HIV and syphilis testing at ANC sites also provided urine samples that were tested for gonorrhoea and chlamydia. The laboratory quality assurance procedures included revalidation of test kits at the time of use with the kit negative and positive control samples; testing all sera for HIV and syphilis by laboratory staff working in Bosaso and Hargeisa reference laboratories as an internal quality control and under supervision of the WHO laboratory services consultant; external quality control was done at Nairobi University Microbiology Department on all sera positive for HIV and syphilis and 10% of negative samples. In Nairobi, HIV tests were done using enzyme-linked immunosorbent assay (ELISA), and ELISA indeterminate samples were tested using western blot.

Results

Using the UAT method, blood samples were collected from 4732 ANC attendees in 13 sites in all the regions. HIV prevalence was determined per site, per zone and for the whole country (both the mean and the median prevalence per zone and for the whole country was calculated).

The HIV prevalence among ANC clinic attendees was 0.9% (the highest was in the north-west: 1.7%), and among TB and STI patients it was 4.5% and 4.3%, respectively. In almost half of the ANC sites, HIV prevalence was higher than 1%. The prevalence of syphilis among ANC attendees was 1.1%.

---

[1] Somalia is divided into three zones: north-west (Somaliland), north-east (Puntland) and south/central zone (Somalia). The country is in a complex emergency situation, with extensive population mobility, low literacy rate and widespread poverty. The population is 9.9 million.

Descriptive data analysis showed that 72% of ANC attendees had had no formal education, 22% had had only primary education and 94% of the total were urban residents. Of these women, 24.6% were attending for the first pregnancy. The highest HIV prevalence was found in the age groups 15–19 and 30–34 years (1.1%), though the women in the age group 44–49 years had prevalence of 2.6% (the total sample for this age group was only 117).

The highest HIV prevalence in TB patients according to age group was found in those aged 35–39 years (6.8%), followed by older than 44 years (5.9%). Among ANC attendees, 0.8% of women were infected with gonorrhoea and 1.7% with chlamydia. Syphilis prevalence among ANC attendees was 1.1%, though in the age group 40–44 years it was 3.1%. Many more women ($n = 1027$) than men ($n = 175$) were included as STI patients, and slightly higher prevalence of HIV was found in men (4.6%) compared to women (4.3%).

Among symptomatic male STI patients, prevalence of gonorrhoea was 1.4% and of chlamydia 2.8%, and no infection was found among women.

Limitations of these surveys

Of note, women included as STI patients were not found to be infected with chlamydia and gonorrhoea, and 2% were found positive for syphilis. The low prevalence of STI in these women is likely to be due to the inclusion of women with reported vaginal discharge, which is largely not due to STI.

Future plans

Somalia is a country now facing a generalized HIV epidemic. Surveillance priorities include conducting probability-based seroprevalence surveys among most-at-risk populations. In addition to FSW, priority populations include displaced persons, lorry drivers, dockworkers, militias, new army recruits, young people and *khat* sellers in Mogadishu, Hargeisa and Bosaso. Another priority is to expand HIV serosurveillance surveys in clinical settings, with data collected regularly every one or two years. Priority areas for conducting community-based seroprevalence surveys will be port towns and larger towns with more developed transportation networks and extensive mobility of population.

Priority ANC sites for close tracking of prevalence and for the provision of prevention of mother-to-child transmission services include Berbera (2.3%), Hargeisa (1.6%) and Gaalkacyo (1.4%). HIV counselling and testing should be offered at all TB and STI clinic sites, with prioritization of those where HIV prevalence in TB and STI patients is highest.

1.2.2 Example of community-based bio-behavioural surveillance in Pakistan

Integrated bio-behavioural surveillance (IBBS) surveys (with HIV and STI testing) were carried out from March to August 2004 in Lahore and Karachi among IDU, FSW and male sex workers, *hijra* and lorry drivers [13]. The study was carried out by the Pakistani Medical Research Council with assistance from Family Health International (FHI).

The sample size per group and per city was 400, except for *hijra*, where the sample size was 200. Biological samples were tested for HIV, syphilis, gonorrhoea and chlamydia, and in women additional tests were done for *Trichomonas vaginalis* and bacterial vaginosis.

Case definitions used for these high-risk populations were the following:

- *female sex workers*: women who have engaged in sex for money as a means of living at least once in the past three months
- *injection drug users*: males who have injected drugs at least once in the past six months
- *male sex workers*: men older than 15 years who had sold sex at least once in the past year
- *hijra*: individuals who were born as males, but have adopted a female sexual personality and dress as women
- *lorry drivers and their assistants*: men driving lorries or assistant drivers along interprovincial transport routes

Sampling included cluster-based sampling of sex workers in Lahore and snowball sampling of sex workers in Karachi. As red-light districts were poorly defined, sampling frame development of venues was difficult. Snowball sampling was also done among male sex workers in Karachi, while in Lahore it was possible to do respondent-driven sampling. Time-location sampling was used to sample IDU in shooting galleries in Lahore and Karachi.

A behavioural questionnaire was completed through face-to-face interview, followed by biological specimen collection (urine, blood). Anal swabs were taken from *hijra* and endocervical swabs from FSW. Treatment was administered for symptomatic STI. All FSW were treated with presumptive therapy for gonorrhoea, chlamydia, trichomonas and bacterial vaginosis as a once-only, and for syphilis according to syndromic management guidelines. Testing took place in Pakistan at the Shaukat Khanum Memorial Cancer Hospital and Research Centre in Lahore and Sindh Institute of Urology and Transplantation in Karachi. The diagnostic tests performed were for HIV (two different ELISAs), syphilis (RPR, TPHA), gonorrhoea (PCR), chlamydia (PCR), bacterial vaginosis (Gram stain), trichomonas (InPouch) and hepatitis C (antibody assay). Participants had access to their HIV test results, deemed necessary by the local health system.

Supervision

A deputy programme manager spent more than 90% of his time in the field supervising and monitoring data collection in Lahore and Karachi.

Main findings

In Karachi, high HIV prevalence was found among IDU (23%), and among male sex workers and *hijra* it was 4% and 2%, respectively. In Lahore HIV prevalence was lower (1% among lorry drivers, and 0.5% among FSW and IDU). Prevalence of gonorrhoea was the highest among FSW (10% in Karachi and 12% in Lahore), as well as chlamydia infection (5% in Karachi and 11% in Lahore). Rectal gonorrhoea was found among 29% of *hijra* and in 18% of male sex workers in Karachi.

Behavioural data showed high frequency of needle-sharing in the week before completion of the questionnaire: 82% in Lahore and 35% in Karachi. Few FSW reported being able to get a condom when needed, and consequently condom use in all recent commercial sex activities was low (2% in Karachi and 19% in Lahore). Other behavioural and biological outcomes from the surveys in Pakistan are described in chapter 5.5.

References

1   *National AIDS programmes: a guide to monitoring and evaluation.* Geneva, UNAIDS, 2000.

2   *Comprehensive plan for epidemiological surveillance.* Atlanta, Georgia, Centers for Disease Control and Prevention, 1986.

3   *Guidelines for second generation HIV surveillance.* Geneva, UNAIDS/WHO, 2000.

4   *Reconciling antenatal clinic-based surveillance and population-based survey estimates of the HIV prevalence in Sub-Saharan Africa.* Geneva, UNAIDS/WHO, 2003.

5   *Guidelines for HIV surveillance among TB patients*, 2nd ed. Geneva, TB/HIV Working Group on the Global Partnership to Stop TB, 2004.

6   Sangani P, Rutherford G, Wilkinson D. Population-based interventions for reducing sexually transmitted infections, including HIV infection. *Cochrane database of systematic reviews*, 2004, 2. At http://www.mrw.interscience.wiley.com/cochrane/clsysrev/articles/cd001220/frame.html.

7   Fleming DT, Wasserheit JN. From epidemiological synergy to public health policy and practice: the contribution of other sexually transmitted diseases to sexual transmission of HIV infection. *Sexually transmitted infections*, 1999, 75(1):3–17.

8   *Report on the global HIV epidemic.* Geneva, UNAIDS/WHO, 2006.

9   *HIV risk behaviour of problem drug users in Greater Cairo.* Geneva, UNAIDS/UNODC, 2004.

10 Draft report. UNAIDS Middle East and North Africa Regional Support Team, 2007.

11 Kaiser R, Kedamo T, Lane J, Kessia G, Downing R, Handzel T, Marum E, Salama P, Mermin J, Brady W, Spiegel P. HIV, syphilis, herpes simplex virus-2 and behavioural surveillance among conflict-affected populations in Yei and Rumbek, southern Sudan. *AIDS*, 2006, 20(6):942–4.

12 Regional database on HIV/AIDS. Cairo, WHO Regional Office for the Eastern Mediterranean.

13 *National study of reproductive tract and sexually transmitted infections.* Survey of high-risk groups in Lahore and Karachi, National AIDS Control Programme. Islamabad, Ministry of Health. Government of Pakistan/Family Health International, 2005.

14 Ministry of Health and Population. HIV/AIDS Biological and Behavioural Survey. Summary report. Egypt 2006. Cairo, Family Health International, 2006.

15 Anderson RM, May RM. *Infectious diseases of humans: dynamics and control.* Oxford, Oxford University Press, 1991.

Part 2

Planning the collection of surveillance information

2.1

Planning for HIV surveillance

Planning for a comprehensive surveillance system at the national level comprises assessment of the HIV epidemic profile and stage and the capacities and structures of the current system, the need for expansion of existing activities to greater geographic coverage or additional populations and the introduction of new methods. This chapter outlines activities for the planning phase of a surveillance system in broad terms and also provides an overview of activities to be conducted in preparation for specific components of surveillance, namely community- and facility-based seroprevalence surveys, described in more detail in subsequent chapters.

The following are key activities in planning for HIV surveillance:

- establishment of an HIV surveillance coordinating committee
- situational assessment of the current HIV epidemic and surveillance system
- definition and prioritization of populations for community-based surveillance surveys
- selection of sites for facility-based surveillance surveys
- determination of the geographical coverage for surveillance activities.

2.1.1 HIV surveillance coordinating committee and surveillance personnel

A multisectoral national surveillance coordinating committee is needed to advise, guide and plan the development of HIV surveillance activities. The surveillance coordinating committee is usually led by the ministry of health or the national AIDS control programme with the inclusion of diverse stakeholder institutions and individuals responding to or affected by the HIV epidemic. These stakeholders include:

- relevant government bodies or ministries (e.g. the ministries of health, youth, education and social affairs)
- other sections of the health system (e.g. public health laboratories, surveillance units for TB and STI, facilities providing HIV care)
- academic institutions and researchers
- international agencies (e.g. WHO, UNAIDS, UNFPA and UNICEF)
- nongovernmental organizations (NGO) that work with most-at-risk populations
- people living with HIV
- other members of civil society affected by the epidemic.

Nongovernmental organizations that work closely with most-at-risk populations can provide unique insight into the needs of the population, where they can be accessed and how programmes can be delivered.

Responsibilities of an HIV surveillance coordinating committee include[1]:

- defining the purpose of surveillance
- identifying data gaps, needs and priority activities
- identifying and selecting priority populations
- prioritizing regions, cities and areas for surveillance activities
- selecting appropriate methods for surveillance
- selecting institutions and experts to provide technical assistance in implementing surveillance activities
- identifying a surveillance coordinator and participation in the selection of project teams for specific surveillance activities
- ensuring that surveillance databases and reports are archived and accessible and that personal information is secure and confidential
- advocating for appropriate levels of funding for surveillance
- ensuring that quality monitoring procedures are implemented
- assisting with data interpretation and the production of an annual surveillance report
- ensuring that surveillance data are disseminated and used for the planning of evidence-based interventions.

While the surveillance coordinating committee has overall responsibility for the above tasks, it may delegate specific tasks to subcommittees or to those overseeing or implementing surveillance activities.

A key position in the implementation of surveillance is the **coordinator**. A coordinator is usually employed by the ministry of health or the national AIDS programme or corresponding body at subnational level. Responsibilities include management and implementation of the national surveillance plan and overseeing implementation of specific surveillance activities.

For each specific component or activity of surveillance, a **project team** is established. Project teams consist of persons with expertise or specific training in epidemiology, data management, statistics, ethnography or anthropology and HIV and STI laboratory methods. Data collection in the field is done by teams with experience in working with the populations at risk for HIV, outreach health education, data collection or abstraction, case management and referral and HIV and STI counselling and testing.

A set of activities with a timeline of implementation for a typical community-based surveillance survey is presented in appendix 2.1.

2.1.2 Situational assessment of the current HIV epidemic and surveillance system

Planning a comprehensive surveillance system requires assessment of the current system's ability to monitor the burden of disease, detect early changes in HIV transmission and

---

[1] Adapted from *The pre-surveillance assessment. Guidelines for planning serosurveillance of HIV, prevalence of sexually transmitted infections and the behavioural components of second generation surveillance of HIV.* Geneva, UNAIDS/WHO Working Group on Global HIV/AIDS and STI Surveillance, 2005.

provide information to develop, target and evaluate the impact of the prevention and care response. The following questions are part of the situational assessment.

- What do we already know about the HIV epidemic?
- What are the results of surveillance activities already in place?
- From the available data, what groups contribute most to the burden of infection in the population and in what geographical areas?
- Are the surveillance system components appropriate to the level of the epidemic in the country? Do they include the groups at highest risk of HIV acquisition and transmission?
- Are there data gaps? What groups at risk are being missed?
- Are surveillance surveys in target groups using standardized sampling methods and data collection instruments that allow comparisons of indicators across areas and over time?
- Is there a need to improve laboratory capacities to more accurately measure HIV and STI prevalence? Are there internal and external laboratory quality assurance procedures in place?
- Is the surveillance system timely enough for the strategic planning cycle?
- Are data used to plan HIV prevention and care activities and to evaluate their impact?
- Is there need for additional resources for HIV surveillance activities?

The situational assessment includes gathering, analysing and interpreting existing data on HIV and STI prevalence, sexual and drug-injecting behaviour, and programme reach and coverage of geographic areas and populations at risk. The purpose of the data review is to find out what is already known about the HIV epidemic. Potential data sources include:

- epidemiological data available from local or national surveillance institutions, including the ministry of health, ministry of education, prison authorities and police
- research publications and reports describing specific aspects of the HIV epidemic in the country available through online databases and journals, such as:
    o PubMed at http://www.ncbi.nlm.nih.gov/entrez/query.fcgi
    o Popline at http://db.jhuccp.org/ics-wpd/popweb/
    o WHO Reproductive Health Library at http://www.rhlibrary.com/
    o *Eastern Mediterranean health journal* at http://www.emro.who.int/emhj.htm
    or at local academic institutions (e.g. masters and doctoral degree theses)
- documents published by international agencies, such as the UNAIDS/WHO Global HIV/AIDS Online Database at http://www.who.int/globalatlas/default.asp
- rapid assessments done by local NGO, government agencies and international organizations
- "grey" literature such as unpublished reports of governmental institutions and NGO
- informal materials from sources such as local magazines, websites, newspapers and guide books (e.g. for mapping locations of high-risk activities).

These documents often contain the names of the local organizations and individuals involved in the response to the HIV epidemic, which in turn help identify key informants and other stakeholders.

The output of the situational assessment should be an archive or comprehensive lists of existing data on the HIV epidemic, a description of the current components and methods of the surveillance system, the organizations involved and the geographical areas and populations covered. This information assists the surveillance coordinating committee to identify data gaps and prioritize the populations for whom more data are needed.

2.1.3 Definition and prioritization of populations for community-based surveillance surveys

Subsequent chapters will describe the methods used to conduct community-based surveillance surveys in most-at-risk populations. This section outlines considerations for defining which most-at-risk populations need to be prioritized at the planning phase.

The definition and prioritization of groups for HIV surveillance activities are guided by trends in HIV and STI prevalence and incidence, the levels and trends in risk behaviour that drive HIV transmission, the ability to take action to intervene with the population and the size of the populations at risk. The following questions may guide selection of priority groups for HIV surveillance.

- Which are most likely to already be infected with HIV? What is the risk behaviour most likely driving HIV transmission?
- Where prevalence is currently low, which groups are most likely soon to be infected with HIV? What behaviour exposes them to HIV?
- What are these groups' potential contributions to the epidemic? What links do they have to other populations?
- What are the sizes of the most-at-risk populations? How mobile are they?
- Are findings from the pre-surveillance assessment and rapid assessment pointing to newly emerging risk groups, new drivers and new areas?

For most areas of the world, the most-at-risk populations have been injection drug users (IDU), female sex workers (FSW) and men who have sex with men (MSM), including male sex workers (MSW). Persons who have sexual contact with members of these groups, e.g. clients of sex workers and spouses of IDU are at elevated risk of exposure to HIV, too. They are included in the bridging populations providing links between most-at-risk populations and the general population. Depending on the sociocultural context in a country bridging populations may include highly mobile populations (e.g. long-distance lorry drivers, fishermen, seafarers and uniformed personnel (e.g. police, military and customs agents).

In planning surveillance in most-at-risk populations, the definitions used need to be based as closely on the consensus of all stakeholders as possible. However, defining the most-at-risk populations nearly always sparks debate. What constitutes an MSM, for example, is highly variable by culture and region. Defining sex work, for example, raises questions of how dependent a person is on sex work as a means of support or how visible the population is. Definitions may be very broad in time frame (e.g. by ever engaging in a particular behaviour) or very specific (currently self-defining as a member of the population). Unfortunately, there are trade-offs in the choice of definitions of the most-at-risk populations that impact HIV surveillance.

On the one hand, definitions of the target groups and inclusion criteria for surveillance surveys (i.e. eligibility criteria and case definitions) should be kept consistent to enable comparison over time and across geographic areas. On the other hand, some persons engaging in the particular risk of interest may not define themselves according to the surveillance case definition and therefore may not be included in surveys. Self-identification is further challenged by stigmatization, laws and taboos related to sexuality and drug use. It is unlikely that there will be universal definitions for most-at-risk populations applicable to all cultures. Nonetheless, we offer the following framework as examples to build on and standardize for specific countries or areas.

Injection drug users

"Current" drug injecting can be defined in many different ways. WHO, UNAIDS and UNODC recommend that for the purpose of measuring indicators for coverage of prevention, care and treatment services, "current" injection drug users should be defined as "persons who have injected any time within the past 12 months" [1]. For the purpose of defining HIV prevalence by mode of transmission, too, this definition or even lifetime injection may be suitable. Some surveillance experts find the definition of current IDU as "persons who have injected drugs during the past two months" useful since it is simple and focuses even more on current injecting behaviour.

"Injectable" drugs are typically thought of as heroin, cocaine and methamfetamine. However, in the recently published WHO multi-site study of HIV/AIDS and injection drug use (WHO Drug Injection Study Phase II), the term "injectable" covered any substance injected outside of a medical context [3].

In order to ascertain drug-injecting behaviour in the course of surveillance activities, survey participants are screened for evidence of recent injecting (e.g. track marks), their ability to describe the process of injecting drugs and for the local cost of drugs. IDU and former IDU can assist with the set of questions that can be used to screen and verify recent injection. Such key informants may be selected from VCT sites, needle exchange programmes and through contacts made by peer educators and former drug users. Typical questions used in the screening process include the following.

- When did you most recently inject drugs?
- What did you most recently inject?
- In which part of your body do you usually inject?
- Can you show me where in your body you most recently injected?
- How much do you usually buy, how is it usually packaged and how much does it cost?

Users of drugs that are not injected are often found to be at elevated risk of HIV infection through increased numbers of sex partners (e.g. exchange of sex for drugs) or impaired ability to negotiate condom use. The definition of non-injection drug use should exclude any lifetime history of injection drug use to make the distinction for the mode of transmission and in the types of prevention intervention needed. Questions included in data collection should include the types of substances used (e.g. opiates, amfetamines, cocaine, crack cocaine, methadone and cannabis) and their frequency of use.

Sex workers

The definition of a sex worker can be highly contentious. On the one hand, public health officials and policy-makers may envision only the most visible types of sex work, such as streetwalkers or brothel-based sex workers (i.e. "direct sex workers") or employees of bars or other entertainment venues who engage in sex work part-time or on the side (i.e. "indirect sex workers"). However, there are many forms of sex work and a vast grey area of exchanging sex for other needs. A typical surveillance definition of a sex worker is someone who has sold sex for money during the past two months when the purpose is to target programmes to current behaviour. Many surveys set the timeframe to the previous year, again with the rationale of the timeframe corresponding to annual surveys.

As with IDU, current or former sex workers can help inform the different types of sex work in the area and help develop screening questions. Such sex workers may be reached through outreach workers and peer educators in bars, streets, brothels or massage parlours. Direct sex workers are likely to be easier to identify in specific venues than indirect sex workers, who may have to be reached through referrals from their networks. In many settings it takes considerable effort and time to establish contacts and trust with sex workers. Screening questions to ascertain the types of sex work include the following.

- When did you most recently exchange sex for drugs, money or other goods?
- Where do you usually find your clients?
- How much money do you get on average from each client?

Men who have sex with men

Men who have sex with men (MSM) exist in all cultures and throughout history. However, the forms that sexual orientation may take are highly variable and elude a single unifying definition. A broad framework for defining sexual orientation incorporates three factors:

- sexual attraction: the degree to which a person is sexually attracted to the same sex
- sexual behaviour: the reported sexual practices engaged in with the same sex
- sexual identity: the words and terms that a person attaches to his or her sexuality.

It may be clear that HIV surveillance is most concerned with sexual behaviour as a mode of HIV transmission rather than attraction or identity. However, particularly in the case of identity, the target population may not be accessed without consideration of how they identify themselves and their networks. Moreover, the potential for future spread of HIV may be affected by a person's level of attraction to the same sex and his or her opportunities for homosexual sex.

A working surveillance definition for MSM would be men who have had sexual activity with other men in the past six or 12 months (men with current homosexual behaviour). As with IDU and sex workers, key informants from the local MSM population can help shape the right screening questions to ascertain if someone meets the surveillance definition. Guiding questions can include the following.

- Do you have sex with men, women or both?
- How often do you have sex with men?
- What types of sex do you engage in with men? Do you engage in receptive anal sex with men? Do you engage in penetrative anal sex with men?

2.1.4 Selection of sites for facility-based surveillance surveys

Some institutions, facilities or clinics include high proportions of most-at-risk populations among their clients and are therefore appealing sites in which to conduct HIV surveillance activities. The methods used should entail minimal disruption of the operations of the facilities, with minimal data collection. Typically, unlinked anonymous HIV testing (UAT) is conducted by using a part of a blood specimen collected for other purposes on a consecutive sample of clients during a specified period of time. This process eliminates biases resulting from declining to participate in HIV testing. WHO and UNAIDS discourage routine testing for HIV without informed consent of the person being tested and promote instead offering a voluntary HIV test routinely to certain clinic populations, e.g. ANC, TB and STI clinic attendees. This approach is known as provider-initiated HIV testing and counselling (PITC). However, in some countries certain facilities may routinely test all clients for HIV, and such data may be used for surveillance purposes if of high enough coverage and good quality. The details of these surveillance methods are provided in subsequent chapters. The present section provides an overview of typical facilities selected for HIV surveillance.

Antenatal clinics

The most common facility for tracking HIV prevalence worldwide has been antenatal clinics (ANC). Pregnant women aged 15 to 49 years are used as proxies to measure the prevalence of HIV in the general sexually active population. ANC HIV prevalence data have been reported routinely to UNAIDS from many countries in the Middle East and North Africa. However, ANC-based HIV surveillance is most appropriate for generalized epidemics and is therefore recommended for the southern part of Sudan, Djibouti and Somalia. Moreover, where ANC HIV prevalence is used as a proxy for national prevalence, data are periodically calibrated against true population-based surveys such as the DHS or AIDS indicator surveys. In countries with generalized HIV epidemics, ANC HIV surveillance is typically conducted every other year with broad geographic coverage of urban and rural areas. In recent years, the increased coverage of provider-initiated HIV testing of pregnant women (e.g. for PMTCT programmes) has raised the possibility of using these programmatic data in place of HIV sentinel surveillance.

However, in low-level and concentrated epidemics such as prevail in most of the Middle East and North Africa, HIV prevalence at ANC may be undetected or of too low a prevalence for meaningful interpretation of levels or trends at ANC. Moreover, very low ANC prevalence cannot be extrapolated to national or regional prevalence without great potential error. As such, for low-level and concentrated epidemics, ANC HIV sentinel surveillance is recommended only in large urban areas or specific areas where HIV prevalence has been documented to exceed 5% in any most-at-risk population. In this manner, ANC sentinel surveillance is serving as a true "sentinel" for the bridging of HIV transmission from most-at-risk populations to the general population—not as a proxy for HIV prevalence in the general population.

The eligibility criteria for inclusion of women in ANC HIV sentinel surveillance typically are:

- attending the clinic during the serosurveillance period for the first time during the current pregnancy

- aged 15–49 years
- acceptance of syphilis testing if HIV testing is carried out using UAT methods.

STI clinics

Because of their shared sexual mode of transmission, patients treated for STI are also at high risk of HIV. Patients seen at STI clinics are therefore a population of great interest to HIV surveillance. STI clinic patients often include a high proportion of most-at-risk populations, such as sex workers and MSM with multiple partners. When screened for and recorded, extra-urethral sites of infection in men (e.g. anal discharge) are strong indicators of male–male sexual behaviour. The methods of conducting facility-based HIV sentinel surveillance at STI clinics are similar to ANC clinics. Eligibility criteria for STI clinic patients include:

- aged 18–59 years
- first visit (i.e. exclude repeat visits)
- presenting with an STI symptom.

This last criterion should be emphasized when the clinic is not exclusively for the diagnosis and treatment of STI, as may typically be the case in the Middle East and North Africa.

Prisons and detention centres

Prisons concentrate many most-at-risk populations, including IDU, other drug users and sex workers. Male prisoners are at higher risk of HIV infection because of possible engagement in male-to-male sex, and for women and men, tattooing and injection drug use while in prison. Sexual violence may also happen to women and men while incarcerated. Surveillance definitions need to consider the length of time in prison to help ascertain if HIV infection was acquired while in the outside community (e.g. included at intake or up to one month) or while incarcerated (i.e. the longer inside increases the probability of infection during incarceration). The use of prisons as HIV sentinel surveillance sites requires close cooperation of prison officials and justice authorities.

Prisoners are appealing populations for HIV prevalence studies by virtue of their fixed location. However, their inclusion in studies and surveillance activities raises special ethical considerations, and established principles in surveillance among prisoners must be followed. *WHO guidelines on HIV infection and AIDS in prisons* states that [1]:

- compulsory testing of prisoners for HIV is unethical
- voluntary testing for HIV infection should be available in prisons when available in the community, with adequate pre- and post-test counselling; voluntary testing should only be carried out with the informed consent of the prisoner
- test results should be communicated to prisoners by health personnel, who should ensure confidentiality
- unlinked anonymous testing for epidemiological surveillance should only be considered if such a method is used in the general population of the country concerned; prisoners should be informed about the existence of any epidemiological surveillance carried out in the prison where they are, and the findings of such surveillance should be made available to the prisoners.

Military and other uniformed personnel barracks or clinics

HIV prevalence among men entering military service is held to reflect HIV prevalence among healthy, sexually active young men in the general population when there is universal conscription (i.e. all young men are required to perform military service). However, in many countries military service is voluntary, and young men of higher socioeconomic classes may avoid it. Police, customs agents and other uniformed personnel in positions of authority are often considered at increased risk of exposure to HIV by virtue of their profession, placing them in contact with sex workers, prisoners and drug users, or by virtue of their mobility and the possibility of multiple sex partners. HIV surveillance data may be collected from samples of uniformed personnel at their barracks or military health clinics

TB clinics

Tuberculosis (TB) is the most common opportunistic infection of people living with HIV worldwide. As such, clinics that treat TB patients are likely to see a comparatively high proportion of HIV-infected persons. HIV surveillance activities can therefore be conducted at TB clinics with a high probability of having measurable HIV prevalence in most epidemic stages. However, it is important to bear in mind that TB is an indicator that the HIV infection may be long-standing and therefore may not be a reflection of the current patterns of HIV transmission in the population. Methods can be UAT or, if HIV testing is universal and routine, through using programmatic data. The eligibility criteria for TB patients for HIV surveillance purposes typically are:

- newly registered
- aged 18–59 years
- acceptance of other blood testing related to TB care if HIV testing is carried out as unlinked anonymous.

Facilities serving migrant and mobile populations

Migrant and mobile men are often considered at increased risk of exposure to HIV by virtue of being separated from their spouses, having sex partners at different locations and isolation from social support. Many migrant and highly mobile men can be accessed either at institutional settings (for example, at the points where they get a work licence or health examination) or can be recruited at sites where they work and socialize (bus stops, sea ports, etc.). Common groups included are:

- long-distance lorry drivers
- construction workers
- fishermen and seafarers
- men who move to major cities for short-term employment.

Migrant and mobile women may also be at elevated risk for HIV infection for similar reasons as men and perhaps for additional reasons as well (vulnerability to sexual violence, exchange of sex for needs). Women who hawk goods along lorry routes in distant towns or across borders, for example, may constitute a vulnerable population.

Programmes for people living with HIV

People living with HIV infection are increasingly recognized as a priority population for targeting HIV prevention programmes—that is, to prevent the onward transmission of infection to others. Indicators to track among people living with HIV include unprotected sex or sharing injection equipment with HIV-negative persons and STI. People living with HIV can be accessed through HIV care clinics.

2.1.5 Determination of the geographical coverage of the HIV surveillance system

In generalized epidemics, surveillance components ideally should scale up to provide national coverage or extensive coverage of the regions where the epidemic is generalized when the pattern is mixed within the country. For example, ANC sentinel surveillance will need to cover rural and urban areas where HIV prevalence has exceeded 1%.

However, in low-level and concentrated epidemics, HIV infections and the populations at risk are usually concentrated in particular areas, such as the capital or other large urban centres or where there is high mobility or migration (e.g. borders, ports, resorts). These areas are likely to have the highest incidence of HIV infection and serve as efficient targets for programme planning. Because there can be large geographical variation in the prevalence of infection, an HIV epidemic in a country may more accurately be conceptualized as a set of different local epidemics at different epidemic stages, rather than as a single national epidemic [4].

Political representation of administrative areas also needs to be taken into consideration when planning the locations of the components of the surveillance system. For example, each region, province or district may require a minimum package of surveillance components, particularly if data are used for the development of region- or district-specific programmes or actions. The following questions raise other considerations for deciding on the geographical coverage of the system.

- Are the surveillance data needed at the national, regional, provincial or district levels?
- To what level do the surveillance data need to be generalized or extrapolated?
- Are there variations in risk behaviour in different parts of the country? For example, do some areas have higher or lower levels of early sexual debut, sex work, mobile men or multiple partners?
- In which areas do the most-at-risk populations congregate and what are their sizes? In which cities or areas does sex work visibly occur? Where are MSM venues more visible? Where is there substantial drug trade?
- Are there cross-border activities with risk groups coming from areas where HIV prevalence is higher, such as mobile populations, involuntary migrants, refugees?
- Where are prevention interventions currently located? Where do they need to be?

2.1.6 Surveillance in complex emergencies

An issue relevant to the Middle East and North Africa is HIV surveillance in complex emergencies, including civil unrest and armed conflict. Such disasters can create large numbers of refugees and internally displaced persons and compromise infrastructure and other health resources. Such conditions may or may not put large numbers of people at higher risk of HIV infection. By international legal definition, **refugees** are persons who are outside their country of nationality and who are unable to return to that country due to fear of persecution. **Internally displaced** people are those who have left their homes due to civil unrest, but have stayed in their country.

Data from many areas of the world present mixed evidence as to whether HIV prevalence among refugees is higher than in their places of origin or their country of refuge, which depends upon the relative prevalence of these locations and the risks refugees incur. Several factors may place refugees and internally displaced persons at higher risk of HIV infection, and therefore warrant high priority for surveillance activities, including:

- sexual interaction of people affected by the emergency with military or paramilitary personnel
- increased economic vulnerability of women and children
- increased frequency of sex work or exchange sex for survival needs
- increased frequency of sexual violence, coercive sex (through manipulation but not the threat of violence) and rape
- increased use of illicit drugs due to psychological trauma and disrupted social networks
- possibility of unsafe blood transfusions
- disrupted preventive and curative services.

2.2

Pre-surveillance and formative assessments

Pre-surveillance activities and formative assessments provide focused information on how to implement a surveillance survey, including choosing appropriate sampling methods, prioritizing the most relevant populations, asking the right questions, gaining access to the populations, establishing relationships with the right gatekeepers and institutions, and field-testing logistics for the planned larger surveillance surveys. For community-based surveillance surveys in most-at-risk populations, ensuring representation of the population depends on the ability to develop a comprehensive sampling frame of sites where target group members congregate (such as for cluster-based sampling and time-location sampling [TLS]) or an in depth understanding of the networks and diversity of a population (such as for respondent-driven sampling [RDS]).

The pre-surveillance assessment is carried out using methods of operational research and can be qualitative and quantitative. The main objectives of the pre-surveillance assessment are:

- to determine, based on known epidemiology and qualitative information, which populations to prioritize for surveillance
- to build alliances between institutions and members of groups at risk for HIV
- to identify potential barriers to surveillance.

The pre-surveillance assessment aims primarily to assess the feasibility of conducting a surveillance survey or activity and to provide information on the surveillance design appropriate to the target population and situation. Pre-surveillance activities specifically seek:

- to determine the feasibility of conducting a surveillance survey, including accessibility of target groups and willingness to participate
- to identify experts, key informants and gatekeepers that can provide information relevant to the implementation of a surveillance survey
- to determine the best possible sampling method for the context and included populations.

After the pre-surveillance, a protocol for the surveillance survey must be finalized. The protocol describes the overall design; procedures and steps of the surveillance survey, including objectives, sampling methods, key measures (biological and behavioural), data management, data analysis and the plan for dissemination; and how the data will be used. A template or outline of such a protocol is given in appendix 2.7. Detailed descriptions of these elements of the protocol can be found in other parts of this book.

2.2.1   Formative assessment in community-based surveillance

Formative assessment done for community-based surveillance relies on many of the tools of qualitative research, such as:

- observation: viewing areas where the target population congregates, observing interactions between members of the population and with others and assessing time periods of high activity and low activity; expansion of observation can include systematic counting or census taking
- creating maps, both physical (e.g. buildings, parks, street locations and neighbourhoods) and ethnographic (e.g. what types of sex worker occur where, what demographic of the target population can be found where)
- focus group discussions: soliciting the diversity and range of issues facing the target population and opinions on methods using a panel of persons from the population or expert in the population
- key informant in-depth interviews: one-on-one interviews with members of the target population or others with unique perspectives on the population or geographic area; building access to the locations where the population congregates and gathering support among the community for the surveillance activities with gatekeepers; pilot-testing the questionnaire for its match to the target population.

The formative assessment for surveillance activities is held to a faster time frame than academic qualitative research with more focused objectives on the information in order to facility the implementation of the surveillance survey itself. Methods resemble those developed for rapid assessment and response (RAR) studies or priorities for local AIDS control efforts (PLACE) (see below). An example of a PLACE study is provided later in this chapter.

In addition to gaining a broad understanding of the target population and how they can be accessed, a specific aim of the formative assessment is to build a qualitative and quantitative framework by identifying the "universe" of points of access (for cluster-based sampling and TLS) and the diversity of the networks of the target populations (for RDS) [6]. The methods of cluster-based sampling, TLS and RDS will be described in detail in subsequent chapters along with other details of the formative assessment specifically accompanying each.

In many settings, places where most-at-risk populations congregate are not easy to find, particularly if such groups are highly stigmatized or their activities are illegal. Such venues might be deliberately hidden, and it can take time to build trust with members of these groups to gain access. Before going into the field, survey coordinators need to enlist gatekeepers and community guides. In addition, if illegal activities are occurring at the sites, authorization from law enforcement will be needed.

Other questions and areas to address during the field assessment include the following.

- Can persons in the selected areas be verified to be engaging in the high-risk behaviour of interest (e.g. is commercial sex happening, are men in the area looking for other men for sex, are the persons hanging out in the area really injection drug users?)
- Is their number large enough to be included in surveillance? For example, in TLS the number may be gauged to be 8 to 10 in a two- to four-hour period minimum to be efficient.
- What is the full range of sites in which the population gathers? To what extent they are difficult to reach at each site? Are persons found at the site networked to others not found at the site?
- Based on the above, what sampling approach is the most appropriate (e.g. cluster-based, TLS, or RDS or non–probability-based methods)?
- Would persons at the sites be willing to answer a behavioural questionnaire and provide biological specimens? If so, what kind of specimens (blood, fingerprick, urine, vaginal, cervical, anal or rectal swab)? What type of incentive would be required for their time?
- What are other factors that affect the conduct of a survey (e.g. safety of staff, transportation, privacy for interviews)?

Pilot-testing of the questionnaire in the formative assessment for clarity, language and comprehension in real field settings helps ensure the questions are in a language understood by target group members in the locations and will be feasible in the field.

During the formative assessment, daily or bi-weekly debriefing sessions should be organized to summarize findings concerning the above questions. In practice, one or a few key informants or periods of observation will not be enough to provide complete information on all venues where members of the priority population can be found. Triangulation of sources is recommended (e.g. using three independent sources such as a community member guide, the police and the venue owner). Ongoing elicitation of venues frequented by members of the most-at-risk population during surveillance activities is also recommended.

For **rds**, the formative assessment specifically explores to what extent target group members are networked with each other and between different subpopulations (e.g. by neighbourhood, demographic characteristics, by behaviour) and their willingness to recruit from their social network for the surveillance survey. Also for RDS, the formative assessment helps the identification of "seeds". The term **seed** refers to initial respondents who will initiate the recruitment of additional respondents through their networks.

For **cluster-based sampling** and **tls**, the formative assessment specifically develops a comprehensive map of the universe of sites or venues where the target population can be found in number. The map serves as the sampling frame for the larger surveillance survey and is discussed in more detail in subsequent chapters. The mapping activities include:

- identifying sites where members of the population congregate, including but not limited to the places where high-risk activities occur or where individuals meet others to then engage in high-risk activities
- assessing the types of high-risk activity (for example, types of sex work, characteristics of clients, patterns of drug use)
- determining what days of the week and times of the day each venue is busiest with members of the most-at-risk population

- counting or estimating the number of target group members present at each location.

Elaboration of the physical map may be done by hand, by writing on paper maps or through GIS software[1]. Physical paper maps may be obtained from local government town planning offices or the national census bureau.

Data collection instruments used in pre-surveillance and formative assessment should have **operational utility** for the purpose of implementation of a surveillance survey. Example forms are provided in the appendix following this chapter.

2.2.2 Formative assessment in facility-based surveillance

In clinic- or facility-based surveillance, the formative assessment focuses on the patient or client population characteristics and operational logistics of the site, including:

- number of clients who visit the facility per day and per month who would meet the surveillance eligibility criteria to estimate the time needed for reaching the sample size
- description of the geographical catchment area
- description of the sociodemographic characteristics of the client population (e.g. age, sex, urban/rural residence)
- routine collection and processing of biological specimens, including quality of the laboratory support (including the equipment available for storage of tests and specimens, time needed for testing and transport of specimens, turnaround for results)
- interest, availability and capacity of staff to participate in data collection
- on-site availability of HIV counselling and testing and referral to services for HIV care
- availability of programmatic data from the same sites (e.g. STI, VCT or PMTCT data).

2.2.3 Team members in formative assessment

Because the formative assessment includes a wide range of activities, members of the team require a diversity of skills and backgrounds, and should include:

- members of the most-at-risk population itself (e.g. MSM, current or former IDU, FSW)
- epidemiologists for secondary data analysis and situational assessment of the HIV epidemic
- experienced research assistants for site observation and enumeration
- ethnographers, anthropologists or others trained in qualitative research methods to conduct key informant interviews, focus group discussions and the analysis of qualitative data.

All staff members who participate in mapping should receive field-based and classroom training before they start the fieldwork. The content of a training workshop should include:

- information on risk groups currently known
- key informant identification and development of rapport

---

[1] Coordinates of venues can be measured using the Global Positioning System (GPS) or hand-written on existing area maps. Some studies have been done using handheld personal digital assistants, which increases efficiency by eliminating data entry and paperwork, and the GPS devices for recording venues' locations (see Mansergh G et al. Adaptation of venue-day-time sampling in south-east Asia to access men who have sex with men for HIV assessment in Bangkok. *Field methods*, 2006, 18[2]:135–52). GPS devices position venues on a world map and allow for assessment of geographical clustering of venues. Mapping can be also done using ArcView mapping software (ESRI Inc. Redlands, California).

- learning how to use the forms that are used in mapping
- communication skills (including interviewing and probing)
- awareness of the sensitive nature of the behaviour that is being explored.

Each field team during data collection should have a supervisor who assigns tasks, handles logistics and maintains quality control.

The team should meet regularly to discuss progress, improve data quality, share experiences and challenges and verify consistency and standardization of methods. A field coordinator assigns the interviewers the number of interviews that they need to complete during a day. They need to receive materials for fieldwork (forms that are provided in appendix 2 or modifications of these forms). Interviewers return completed questionnaires at the end of each day and receive instructions from a coordinator for the next day.

A sampling frame for groups at high risk of HIV is developed for a specific geographical area, and therefore the results cannot be generalized at the national level. Hence, results of the pre-surveillance assessment and mapping are representative for that population subgroup and a particular geographical area only. Detailed guidance on how to do mapping of venues is described in the PLACE method manual, which is available at https://www.cpc.unc.edu/measure/leadership/place.html. Additional information on methods of rapid assessment can be found in *Technical guide to rapid assessment and response (TG-RAR)*. Geneva, WHO, 2003. Available at http://www.who.int/docstore/HIV/Core/Index.html; and also in Fitch C, Stimson GV. *A report from the WHO drug injection study phase II*. Geneva, WHO, 2003. Available at http://www.who.int/substance_abuse/activities/drug_injecting/en/.

More on how to conduct focus groups for the purposes of HIV-related formative research can be found in the following.

Mack N, Woodsong N, MacQueen KM, Guest G, Namey E. *Qualitative research methods: a data collector's field guide*. Arlington, Virginia, USAID/Family Health International, 2005.

Wilson D. *HIV/AIDS rapid assessment guide by Family Health International*. Arlington, Virginia, USAID/Family Health International, 2001. Available at http://www.fhi.org/en/HIVAIDS/pub/guide/HIV_Rapid_Assessment_Guide.htm.

Lambert EY, Ashery RS, Needle RH, eds. *Qualitative methods in drug abuse and HIV research*. Rockville, Maryland, National Institute of Health, 1995. National Institute on Drug Use Research Monograph 157. Available at http://www.drugabuse.gov/pdf/monographs/download157.html.

2.2.4   Example of a formative assessment with mapping in Pakistan

Mapping was done to develop sampling frames for surveillance surveys of sex workers in Karachi and Rawalpindi, Pakistan, through mapping and enumeration.

Geographical distribution of the target area

The areas under study were divided geographically into smaller data collection units. In Karachi, zones were made based on the administrative divisions of the city while in Rawalpindi physical landmarks were used to divide the city into several zones. Based on experience from pilot studies, existing administrative divisions called union councils were found to be an effective way to demarcate zones into manageable subunits. Two to four union councils were combined to form one zone.

The mapping activities were divided into two levels (level 1 and level 2).

Level 1 activities

Level 1 focused on collecting information about most-at-risk populations in various geographical locations in each zone and recording information on forms.

Key informants were selected from respected and well connected members of the areas who were expected to provide information on the areas and estimates of the number of most-at-risk populations members present[1]. Identifying areas where high-risk activities took place was the first step in data collection. Experience showed that 20–30 interviews in each zone (two to four union councils) delivered sufficient information judged by their consistency and saturation (i.e. no new information was obtained with more interviews).

Emphasis was placed on providing estimated numbers (minimum and maximum) of most-at-risk populations members for each location or specific spot through interviews with key informants. For instance, a key informant may have reported that there were 10–15 home-based female sex workers in a certain spot. Ten was then taken as the minimum estimate and 15 as the maximum estimate for that particular interview.

In addition to collecting information on most-at-risk populations, a list of contact persons at various locations who could provide further information on high-risk activities was also developed. These persons provided a link to high-risk individuals for level 2 activities.

Data collation

After field activities, the field team assembled to collate the data collected on a daily basis. Data were edited by sorting information into tables and electronic databases.

---

[1]   **Key informants** were defined in this study as persons who were likely to have information about the locations and number of participants involved in high-risk activity. Based on their involvement with high-risk activities and most-at-risk populations, key informants were classified into three types:
  1. primary key informants: persons engaged in risk activities themselves (e.g. commercial sex workers and injection drug users)
  2. secondary key informants: persons who were involved in the network of risk activities or intimately acquainted with persons directly engaged in risk activities (e.g. pimps and taxi drivers)
  3. tertiary key informants: persons involved with high-risk activities in a professional capacity (e.g. police, STI service providers and nongovernmental organization workers).

The first step of data collation involved consolidation of the places reported in level 1 interviews, based on the number of times they were mentioned by different key informants (this is referred to as **frequency of mention**). The final estimates of the population size at each place were prepared by collating minimum and maximum estimates. All spots that were identified during data collection were marked on the city map. A table was made with all the sites mentioned and formed the basis for selection of places to visit in level 2 activities.

Level 2 activities

The focus of the level 2 activities was to validate the data from level 1 activities and to conduct interviews to solicit information on:

- activities at the place related to risk behaviour (e.g. looking for sex partners, clients or drugs) and taking risks (places where sexual acts or injecting drugs occur)
- the number of sex workers
- the average number of clients of each sex worker at each place
- information about network operators
- information about STI service providers and health services.

The final step in data collection involved conducting interviews with key informants at places within all identified locations in each zone. This activity served as a verification step of data collected during level 1.

At least three places (ideally the three with the highest number of key informants) in each zone were visited, and three interviews with primary key informants were conducted at each spot. If primary key informants were not available, secondary key informants were used.

Data collected in this manner were systematically extrapolated to the two cities and elsewhere to assist with estimating the number of sex workers in Pakistan. The mapping also provided the sampling frame for community-based surveillance surveys.

2.3

Ancillary surveillance activities

2.3.1 Estimating the size of the populations at risk

Although surveys and other surveillance activities to determine prevalence of HIV and risk behaviour can be conducted on hidden populations without knowing their true numbers, the data generated will be limited in interpretation and use unless an estimate of the population size is available. For example, projected numbers of new HIV infections, the coverage of interventions and programmes and appropriate resource allocation cannot be done effectively without knowing how many persons there are in the population at risk and being served. For example, if the target of a harm reduction intervention is to provide 70% of IDU with sterile needles, data are needed on how many injectors there are for the purchase and distribution of injection equipment. Knowing the size of most-at-risk populations also helps assess whether the desired sample size can be reached in community-based surveillance surveys, particularly when the population is small or the location is a small town.

While surveillance surveys in themselves do not estimate the size of the most-at-risk population, they can be efficiently combined with other methods of estimation with proper planning and coordination. Some methods can be conducted with the formative phase (e.g. mapping and enumeration); other methods entail the addition of questions to the survey questionnaire (e.g. multipliers, population-based surveys); other methods entail intercepting the target population before or after the surveillance survey (e.g. capture–recapture). Data from surveillance surveys also assist in extrapolation of local estimates to the national level.

The formative assessment phase of a surveillance survey can also provide counts or estimates for certain components of the population of interest using existing secondary data sources, for example:

- registries of drug users in treatment programmes provide counts for part of the IDU population
- police data provide counts of parts of the sex worker and drug-user population arrested
- prison data provide the current number of prisoners
- data from outreach programmes of nongovernmental organizations may count the number of clients they serve
- clinic or hospital data counts of drug-related admissions, overdoses, wound infections, HIV-infected IDU, etc.

- data from needle exchange programmes may count clients served
- union and employment data provide counts of some occupations (e.g. lorry drivers, seafarers).

These sources in and of themselves do not provide a complete count of the population; however, they can provide lower limit estimates and a basis for other methods of estimation (e.g. multiplier methods).

Service-based data sources in themselves have several limitations in counting the size of the most-at-risk population. It may not be possible to distinguish who are actual members of the most-at-risk population. For example, VCT sites may not record if clients are MSM or FSW, or such information may not be disclosed by clients. Moreover, services are often only used by a small fraction of the total members of the most-at-risk population. However, counts provided by service data may be used to extrapolate to the whole most-at-risk population when combined with community-based surveys, as discussed below.

The following describes several methods to estimate the size of hidden or hard-to-reach populations which can be combined with surveillance surveys. These are based on the UNAIDS publication *Estimating the size of the populations at risk for HIV*, where also more detailed descriptions can be found [11]. Additional information on population size estimation may be found in a supplement to the journal *Sexually transmitted infections* (2006, 82[supplement 3]).

Mapping, census and enumeration methods

The mapping conducted for the formative assessment for surveillance can be expanded to produce a systematic count (i.e. census) of the population of interest within the mapped area, for example, of FSW in a city. Once all areas where sex work occurs have been identified, enumeration or counting of the women engaging in sex work in each area is made. Standardized rules are set to avoid duplication (e.g. by using the same guides and staff in a given area) and undercounting (e.g. by appearing on several different days and times). The enumeration may be based on the responses of key informants (as described in the example from Pakistan above) or by direct counting by field staff. When the venues are numerous, a random or systematic sample can be taken and the average number present can be applied to the universe of venues (e.g. an average of 50 women per brothel times 25 brothels in the city). Averages and rates per areas or cities may then be used to extrapolate to wider regions or the country. Mapping, census and enumeration methods are more appropriate for visible target groups, populations that are not widely scattered or found in fixed locations.

Population-based surveys

The implementation of population-based surveys used for multiple purposes including HIV surveillance, such as the demographic and health surveys or AIDS indicator surveys, provides an opportunity to produce an estimate of populations at risk in a nationally representative sample [12]. For example, many such surveys ask questions on exchange of money or other goods for sex. In surveys of many industrialized countries, such as the National Survey of Sexual Health and Attitudes in the United Kingdom, questions are included to estimate the number of MSM by asking the sex of sexual partners in the past five years [13]. Population size estimates are calculated by applying the prevalence in the survey sample to the overall number of people living in a country or an area. However, such surveys are likely to underestimate the number of people who engage in high-risk activities due to severe stigma and the illegal nature of some behaviour (including sex work, drug use and male–male sex in many areas of the Middle East and North Africa). Moreover, even with sincere answers to such questions, the numbers are likely to be small and therefore imprecise.

Multiplier methods

An appealing and relatively low-cost method to estimate the size of the most-at-risk population is the multiplier method. This method uses data from two sources and examination of the overlap between the two sources, including an unduplicated count of members of the most-at-risk population from an independent list (e.g. number of FSW receiving a particular service from an NGO in a defined time period in a defined location) and the insertion of a question on the use of the specific service into a community survey instrument.

For example, IDU can be asked whether they were in public detoxification treatment during the previous year in the community-based surveillance survey. In this scenario the ministry of health knows that there were 1000 IDU in treatment during the previous year. If 30% of IDU said that they were in this treatment programme in the previous year, then the total population size can be estimated as 1000/0.30 = 3333 IDU in that city.

The multiplier method based on use of services estimates only the size of the population at a very local level. Several multipliers can be used simultaneously to strengthen the rigour of the estimate (e.g. producing a median estimate and range). The choice of multipliers is determined by the availability and quality of the unduplicated count available in each location during the formative phase of the project. The survey questions need specifically to identify the services in question and the specific time period. For example, in an RDS among FSW, participants would be asked which specific services or sites (e.g. VCT, STI, prison) they have visited in a specific time period (e.g. past 12 months). The next step entails collecting unduplicated counts of FSW clients who were seen for services in the past 12 months at the specific sites mentioned in the survey.

Although apparently simple, the multiplier method has many limitations that may result in biased estimates of the population size. These include non-independence of participants in the survey and the services (i.e. the same persons are more likely to be in both resulting in underestimation), lack of identification as a member of the target population in the service data (resulting in overestimation), inability to unduplicate individuals seen multiple times at the service (producing overestimation).

Capture-recapture

The capture-recapture method has existed for centuries and has been used in zoology (e.g. to estimate the number of fish in a lake). It has come into wider use for estimating hidden populations of people with AIDS [14, 15, 16, 17]. The principle of capture-recapture resembles the multiplier method in that two sources of data are needed, in this case, two independent samples of the target population. The population size estimate is given the number of persons of the population "captured" (recruited) in each survey and the number in both using the formula:

$$N = \frac{n_1 n_2}{m}$$

where N is the total population size; n_1 is the number recruited into the first survey; n_2 the number recruited into the second; and m is the number "recaptured" in both surveys. The 95% confidence interval is given by:

$$95\% \text{ CI} = N \pm 1.96\sqrt{\text{Var } (N)} \text{ ; where Var } (N) = \frac{n_1 n_2 (n_1 - m)(n_2 - m)}{m^3}$$

Four underlying assumptions or criteria must be met to use the capture-recapture method:

- the samples must be independent of one another (i.e. not correlated)
- each member of the population should have an equal, non-zero probability of being "captured" and "recaptured"
- the individuals identified in both captures must be correctly identified, and no one else should wrongly be identified as a recapture
- there should be no major immigration or out-migration from the population between the initial and the second captures.

It is rare that the four conditions for reliable capture-recapture estimates are perfectly met in populations at high risk of HIV.

Example of population size estimation for injection drug users in Tolyatti, Russia: implications for harm reduction and coverage

The aim of this study, carried out in 2001, was to estimate the prevalence of IDU in Tolyatti, Russia, and to examine the implications of these estimates for harm reduction programmes. The multiple sample capture-recapture method was used examining the multiple overlaps of individual IDU in three programmatic data sources. The approach estimated the size of the IDU population and further gauged the coverage of the programmes.

Methods

Available routine programmatic data sources of IDU were identified, and individuals were matched across the sources using sex, year of birth, initials of first name and surname and district of residence to identify subjects in only one, two or three data sources. Only exact matches were used on the following three data sources: HIV-positive test results recorded at the AIDS centre (n = 1355); IDU registered at a narcology service (n = 3980); and police arrest data on individuals arrested for the possession of illegal drugs or drug-injecting equipment (n = 2806). Of note, many IDU are arrested for offences other than drug possession, including sex work and theft; this factor will result in underestimation. Other data sources were attempted, such as emergency room overdose admissions and STI clinic records; however, IDU status was not collected or the complete data were not available for matching. Although the police arrest data did not record whether an individual was an IDU, it was assumed that all subjects arrested for small quantities of injectable drugs (heroin and home-produced opiates or amfetamines) were classified as IDU. Analysis was conducted on those aged 15–44 years and resident in the city. Population estimates were calculated for two groups: the officially registered IDU population, excluding migrants; and population estimates that included migrants.

As a multiple sample recapture, Poisson regression or log–linear models are fitted to the observed data, with interactions between data sources fitted to replicate "dependencies" between those data sources to adjust for this bias. The best-fitting model was used to estimate the number of injection drug users "not observed" in any data sources, and thereby estimate the overall prevalence of injection drug use in the overall population of the city.

Results

In total, there were 8141 records identified as IDU from the three data sources: AIDS centre (n = 1355); narcology service (n = 3980); police arrest data (n = 2806) with 5222 individual IDU identified after matching. The police data source "captured" proportionally more males and older IDU than the other data sources. In total, 1104 (21%) of the sample were matched in more than one data source and 80 (2%) were matched in all three data sources.

Based on these data, the total number of IDU in Tolyatti was estimated to be 20 226 (range 16 971–24 749) giving a population prevalence of 5.4% (range 4.5%–6.6%) of the city population and 2.8% (range 2.4%–3.5%) for the unregistered IDU population aged 15–44 years using a Poisson model.

Of note, there was less overlap within the data sources for female compared to male IDU; only one matched record for females was found in all three data sources in the 15–24 age group and one between 25 and 44 years. Such small overlaps will result in more imprecision in the estimates for female IDU. For comparison of the ratio of male to female IDU, data from emergency rooms indicate a ratio of 7:1 men to women presenting for opiate overdose during 2001. The only routine data in Tolyatti that indicated an equal ratio between men and women are the data from outreach monitoring, which reported a ratio of 1:1.3 men to women.

2.3.2 Priorities for local AIDS control efforts (PLACE) and other rapid assessment approaches

Because PLACE emphasizes public health action in a very specific location, it cannot be generalized and therefore may not be considered a routine component of HIV surveillance. Nonetheless, the tools used in PLACE very much resemble those of the pre-surveillance and formative assessment for community-based surveillance surveys [7].

PLACE employs detailed mapping, key informant interviews, focus group discussions, observation and rapid convenience sample surveys in small areas where high-risk groups gather and where high-risk behaviour itself may occur (i.e. "hotspots"). Examples include lorry stops where commercial sex work is very common, areas of specific economic activity (e.g. mines, plantations, markets) or areas of much drug selling, buying and use.

The PLACE method identifies and maps public venues where people engage in high-risk behaviour and estimates the extent of new partnership formation, sexual mixing and drug use among the population socializing at these venues [8]. Subsequently, it provides information to local intervention planners about where to reach individuals most likely to acquire and transmit HIV and what types of intervention are needed. A final phase may evaluate the actions by reassessing risk and programme coverage after a period of time. Rather than simply describing individuals, PLACE defines the target population based on attendance at venues rather than based on membership of a risk group or occupation.

A strength of PLACE is that it facilitates rapid development and implementation of venue-specific prevention programmes. A complete PLACE manual with example data collection forms can be downloaded from https://www.cpc.unc.edu/measure/leadership/place.html. Similar forms have been adapted for the purpose of the more focused pre-surveillance assessment and are available in appendixes 2.1–2.5.

Appendix 2

The forms for the pre-surveillance assessment can be modified by adding questions that are important for the local pre-surveillance activities

---

[1] Data collection forms 2.2–2.4 are adapted from: *PLACE: priorities for local AIDS control efforts. A manual for implementing the PLACE method.* Chapel Hill, North Carolina, Measure evaluation, 2005.

Appendix 2.1

Timeline for planning of the surveillance survey

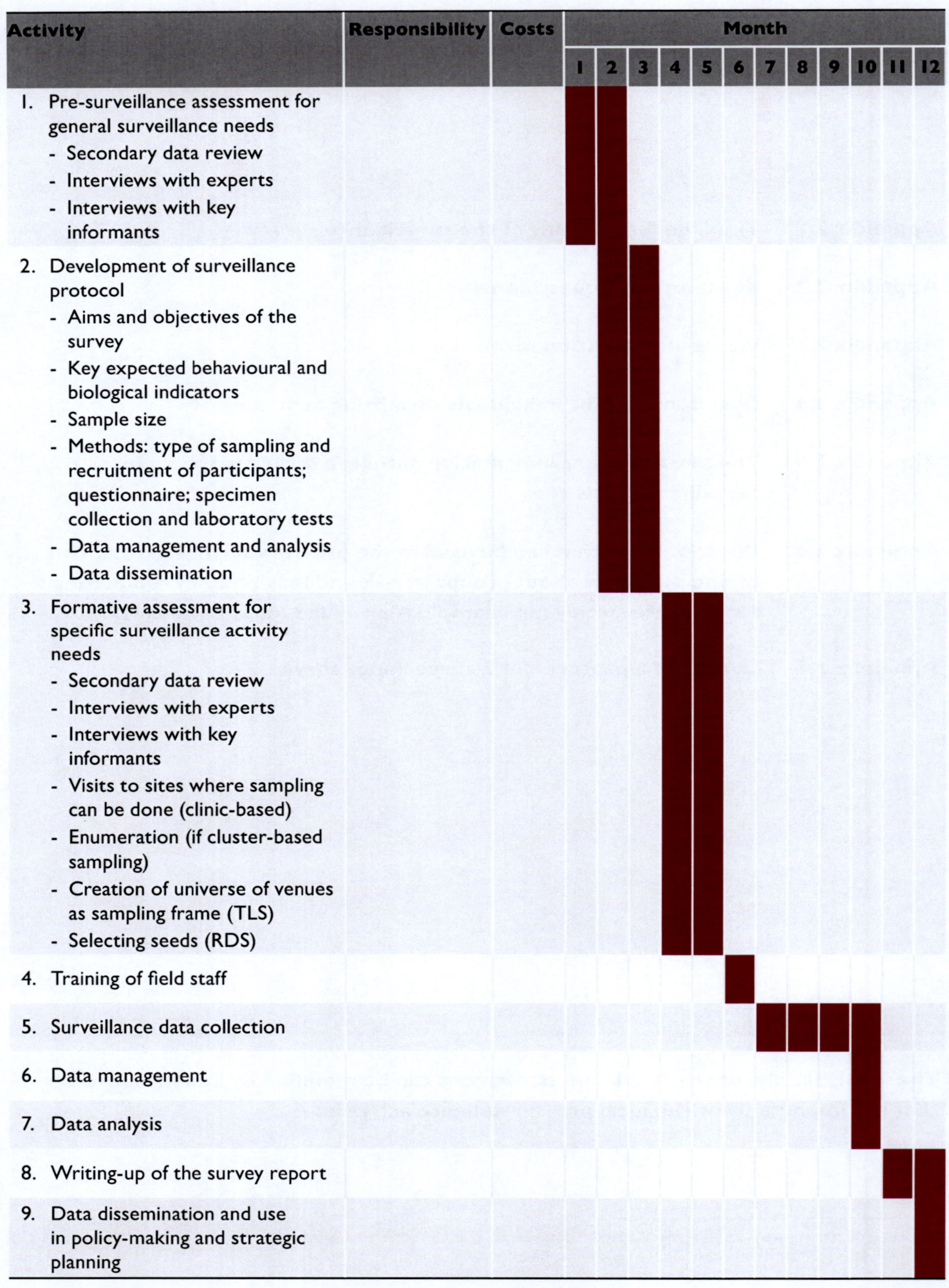

Activity	Responsibility	Costs	Month											
			1	2	3	4	5	6	7	8	9	10	11	12
1. Pre-surveillance assessment for general surveillance needs - Secondary data review - Interviews with experts - Interviews with key informants			■	■										
2. Development of surveillance protocol - Aims and objectives of the survey - Key expected behavioural and biological indicators - Sample size - Methods: type of sampling and recruitment of participants; questionnaire; specimen collection and laboratory tests - Data management and analysis - Data dissemination				■	■									
3. Formative assessment for specific surveillance activity needs - Secondary data review - Interviews with experts - Interviews with key informants - Visits to sites where sampling can be done (clinic-based) - Enumeration (if cluster-based sampling) - Creation of universe of venues as sampling frame (TLS) - Selecting seeds (RDS)						■	■							
4. Training of field staff									■					
5. Surveillance data collection										■	■	■		
6. Data management												■		
7. Data analysis													■	
8. Writing-up of the survey report													■	
9. Data dissemination and use in policy-making and strategic planning														■

Appendix 2.2

Key informant questionnaire

This is sample of a data entry sheet that can be used during the process of mapping locations where members of most-at-risk populations congregate. It is done by asking key informants about venues where high-risk activities take place. These venues are places where people meet new commercial sex partners, exchange drugs for money, etc.

Q1	Interviewer name	
Q2	Name of location	
Q3	Date of data collection	(dd/mm/yy) ___________| ___________| ___________|
Q4	Address	
Q5	Key informant number	
Q6	Sex of key informant	
Q7	Age of key informant	
Q8	Type of key informant	e.g. gatekeeper, police officer, member of most-at-risk population
Q9	Can you tell me where /here state which target group/ go to spend time or hang out to find partners/ drugs, etc.?	
Q10	How would you describe the population of /here state which target group/ in the local area, in terms of their age and socioeconomic status?	

Appendix 2.3

Venue verification form

This form is used after the form in appendix 2.2 and is filled out at the venue. It is used in mapping activities at the venue by collecting information from key informants and target group members. It is done as part of mapping and preparations for sampling.

Q1	Unique venue number	
Q2	Address of the venue	
Q3	Date of interview	(dd/mm/yy) ________	________	________	
Q4	How many informants reported that venue?	
Q5	Was the venue found?	01. Yes and venue in operation 02. Yes but venue closed temporarily 03. Venue closed permanently 04. Address insufficient, venue not found 05. Duplicate venue
Q6	Type of venue[1]	
Q7	Number of respondents (and/or code)	
Q8	Sex of respondent	
Q9	Type of respondent[2]	
Q10	Age of respondent	
Q11	What types of activity take place at the venue?	01. Men meet new female sex partners 02. Women meet new sex partners 03. Female sex workers solicit customers 04. Men meet male sex partners 05. MSM socialize 06. Buying drugs. If so, what type of drugs? 07. Injecting drugs
Q12:	What are the busiest times in the year at the venue (by month)?	

---

[1] The types of venue can be:
eating/drinking/dancing places: informal bars, formal bars, nightclubs, massage parlours, brothels, hotels, hostels, overnight lorry stops, other.
transportation/public/commercial areas: bus or train stations, lorry stops, taxi stands, ports, beaches, streets or street corners, parks, markets, school or university neighbourhoods, stores, shopping centres, tourist attractions, other.
[2] Can be bar owner, staff, member of the target group of interest, etc.

Q13	What are the busiest times of the month at the venue?				
Q14	How many people who are target group members[1] attend the venue during a week and during the specified times. Write down in the table the number of men and women found at the venue. The time-periods can be broken down to smaller units (for example, from 6 pm to 8 pm).	**Morning** **6 am–noon**	**Afternoon** **noon–6 pm**	**Evening** **6 pm–10 pm**	**Late night** **10 pm–6 am**
		Monday			
		Tuesday			
		Wednesday			
		Thursday			
		Friday			
		Saturday			
		Sunday			
Q15	Are there any particular recruitment barriers, such as large number of people, unfriendly management, or problems with safety?				
Q16	What do you think would motivate people to participate in the survey?				
Q17	What should we *not* do or *not* say as part of our recruitment effort?				
Q18	Who else do you know might be particularly good at helping to understand better where and how to conduct the survey?				
Q19	Do you have any other recommendations?				

---

[1] Or who undertake high-risk activities.

Appendix 2.4

Questionnaire for individuals socializing at venues

This form can be used at the same time as the form in appendix 2.3. It is used for interviewing people who engage in high-risk activities and who are found at the venue.

Q1	Unique venue number	
Q2	Address of the venue	
Q3	Date of interview	(dd/mm/yy) _________ | _________ | _________ |
Q4	Type of venue	
Q5	Number of respondent (and/or code)	
Q6	Sex of respondent	
Q7	How often do you come here?	
Q8	Why did you come here?	01. To socialize 02. To drink alcohol 03. To look for a sex partner 04. To buy drugs 05. To work 06. Something else (specify)
Q9	How many other places have you been today to socialize, drink alcohol or look for a sex partner? Please specify the names of the places	
Q10	How many other places do you plan to visit today to socialize, drink alcohol or look for a sex partner? Please specify the names of the places	

Q11	Have you ever had sex with a person you first met here?
Q12	Have you given or received money in exchange for sex in the past four weeks?
Q13	Have you given or received money in exchange for sex in the past 12 months?
Q14	In your opinion, do people who use drugs socialize at this site?
Q15	In your opinion, do people who inject drugs socialize at this site?
Q16	In your opinion, can drugs be bought here?

Appendix 2.5

The most relevant information gathered during mapping for surveillance activities

The following table can be used at the end of mapping to list the number of target group members found at each venue. List each two-hour time period when approximately four population members can be surveyed. The information on line 1 is an example of the type of data entered in each field.

No.	Venue name	Location	Types of risk activity	SUN	MON	TUE	WED	THUR	FRI	SAT	Safe (yes/no)	Number of eligible respondents during a two-hour period
1	Mix	North side, bus station		2p – 4p	8p – 10p	8p – 10p	8p – 10p	8p – 10p	9–11p 12–1a	9–11p 12–1a		
2												
3												
4												
5												
6												
7												
8												
9												
10												
11												
12												

Appendix 2.6

Questionnaire that can be used in pre-surveillance assessment to find out more about groups at risk and feasibility of conducting a surveillance survey

An example is provided for sex workers. The questionnaire consists of open-ended and closed questions.

<table>
<tr><td colspan="2">Name of interviewer</td></tr>
<tr><td colspan="2">Date of interview</td><td>(dd/mm/yy) _________ | _________ | _________ |</td></tr>
<tr><td colspan="2">Where is the interview being conducted?</td></tr>
<tr><td>I.</td><td colspan="2">SCREENING QUESTION[1]
(TO ESTABLISH WHETHER SOMEONE IS A SEX WORKER)</td></tr>
<tr><td>1.1</td><td colspan="2">When was the last time you sold sex for money or goods?</td></tr>
<tr><td>1.2</td><td colspan="2">How much do you charge?</td></tr>
<tr><td>2.</td><td colspan="2">DEMOGRAPHIC QUESTIONS</td></tr>
<tr><td>2.1</td><td colspan="2">What year were you born?</td></tr>
<tr><td>2.2</td><td colspan="2">Your marital status is: single ☐ married ☐ divorced ☐ widowed ☐</td></tr>
<tr><td>2.3</td><td colspan="2">What kind of education do you have: none[2] ☐ primary ☐ secondary ☐ tertiary ☐</td></tr>
<tr><td>2.4</td><td colspan="2">How long have you been living in this city/area?</td></tr>
<tr><td>3.</td><td colspan="2">QUESTIONS ON THE NATURE OF THE SEX WORK</td></tr>
<tr><td>3.1</td><td colspan="2">Can you describe what kinds of sex work exist in the city/area (brothels, street, saunas, flats, other?)</td></tr>
<tr><td>3.2</td><td colspan="2">Where are these sites where sex work happens?</td></tr>
<tr><td>3.3</td><td colspan="2">What is the age range of women/men who engage in sex work?</td></tr>
<tr><td>3.4</td><td colspan="2">Are there women from other countries or any ethnic minority women that work as sex workers? If so, where do they come from?</td></tr>
<tr><td>3.5</td><td colspan="2">Are any of the women using drugs? If so, what type of drugs? Do they inject?</td></tr>
</table>

---

[1] Before going to the questions, a rapport needs to be built with each interviewee by describing the purpose of the study and stressing the anonymity and confidentiality of interviewing. This is particularly important if we expect good-quality answers on open-ended questions. After this introduction, a participant can be asked to give informed oral consent.

[2] If none, ask whether she/he can read and write.

3.6	Are there any men that sell sex that you know of?	
4.	**QUESTIONS ON THE INTERVIEWEE'S OWN EXPERIENCE AS A SEX WORKER**	
4.1	Which part(s) of the city do you work in?	
4.2	Have you been working anywhere else before? If yes, where?	
5.	**QUESTIONS RELATED TO THE FEASIBILITY OF COLLECTING BIOLOGICAL SPECIMENS**	
5.1	Would you be willing to give blood for an HIV test, which will be anonymous and confidential, for a study that aims to identify better health programmes that are needed in this area in order to prevent the spread of diseases that are transmitted by sex?	
5.2	Do you think that other sex workers that you know would be willing to give blood for an HIV test?	
5.3	Would you be willing to get tested for sexually transmitted infections by giving urine or by a doctor examining you (performing a genital examination)?	
6.	**QUESTIONS FOR EXPLORING THE FEASIBILITY OF CONDUCTING SURVEILLANCE SURVEYS**	
6.1	Can you please tell me more about the sites where you think sex workers gather in the city/area and where they seek their clients?	
6.2	How many other sex workers do you know by name who know you? Do they live in the same area/city, and have you seen them in the past three months?[1, 2]	
6.3	Do you do any activities with other sex workers like going out, shopping or other forms of socializing?	
6.4	Would you be willing to participate in this study for free?[3] If not, would you be willing to participate if you received food, money, etc.?	

---

[1]   This period can be longer or shorter, depending on the findings from the formative research.
[2]   This question is asked to find out about the feasibility of conducting respondent-driven sampling. However, other questions also need to be asked (see section 3.4 in the guidelines).
[3]   Here mention what the benefits of participation are.

Appendix 2.7

Outline of a protocol for a surveillance survey

The surveillance protocol is written by the principal investigator for each surveillance survey and serves as a guide to all staff who work on the survey. The protocol development process also includes development of a budget since available financial resources can affect survey design. The protocol contains sections that are described in more detail elsewhere in the guidelines, and its precise content will depend on the design of the surveillance survey and other operational and logistical issues.

The protocol should consist of the following elements.

1. Aim and objectives of the surveillance survey

2. Roles of implementing agencies

3. Description of the formative research

4. A justification for the selection of the target group and geographic locations for surveillance and the frequency with which the surveillance survey will take place

5. Training of staff

6. Sample size requirements

7. Methods:
   - operational definitions of the target group
   - key indicators that will be obtained, including biological and behavioural, and outcome and impact indicators
   - sampling approach
   - development and validation of tools and instruments
   - testing on HIV, STI and parenterally acquired infections
   - selection and training of interviewers, supervisors, data entry clerks, laboratory staff
   - data collection procedures
   - quality control

8. Any interventions provided (pre- and post-test counselling, educational materials, case management)

9. Compensation for participation (if required)

10. Ethics of the survey (how anonymity and confidentiality will be safeguarded)

11. Data management

12. Data analysis

13. Writing of surveillance reports, which should include the following sections:
    - aims and objectives
    - methods
    - results (behavioural and biological indicators)
    - interpretation of data with discussion
    - limitations of the survey
    - relevance of the survey for planning of HIV prevention efforts and future surveillance
    - suggested interventions that need to be undertaken based on the results

14. Dissemination of results

15. Budget

References

1   *WHO/UNODC/UNAIDS technical guide for countries to set targets for universal access
    to HIV prevention, treatment and care for injecting drug users (IDUs)*. Geneva, WHO,
    2009.

2   Des Jarlais DC, Perlis TE, Stimson GV, Poznyak V, the WHO Phase II Drug
    Injection Collaborative Study Group. Using standardized methods for research on
    HIV and injecting drug use in developing/transitional countries: case study from the
    WHO Drug Injection Study Phase II. *BMC public health*, 2006, 6:54.

3   Fitch C, Stimson GV. A report from the WHO Drug Injection Study Part II. RAR-
    Review. *An international review of rapid assessments conducted on drug use*. Geneva,
    WHO, 2003.

4   Wasserheit JN, Aral SO. The dynamic topology of sexually transmitted disease
    epidemics: implications for prevention strategies. *Journal of infectious diseases*, 1996,
    174(suppl 2):S201–13.

5   Higgins DL, O'Reilly K, Tashima N, Crain C, Beeker C, Goldbaum G, Elifson
    CS, Galavotti C, Guenther-Grey C. Using formative research to lay the foundation
    for community level HIV prevention efforts: an example from the AIDS Community
    Demonstration Projects. *Public health report*, 1996, 111(suppl):28–35.

6   McFarland W, Caceres C. HIV surveillance among men who have sex with men.
    AIDS, 2001, 15(suppl 3):S23–32.

7   Weir SS, Tate J, Hileman SB, Khan M, Jackson E, Johnston A, Herman C.
    Priorities for local AIDS control efforts. A manual for implementing the PLACE method.
    Chapel Hill, North Carolina, Carolina Population Center, Measure Evaluation,
    2005. At http://www.cpc.unc.edu/measure/leadership/place.html.

8   Weir SS, Tate JE, Zhusupov B, Boerma JT. Where the action is: monitoring local
    trends in sexual behaviour. *Sexually transmitted infections*, 2004, 80(suppl 2):ii63–8.

9   Stover J. New approaches to effectively programming HIV/AIDS prevention
    resources. *Bulletin of the World Health Organization*, 2005, 83(5):383.

10 *A situational analysis guide on sex work in west and central Africa*. Washington DC,
    World Bank/UNAIDS, 2000.

11 Pisani E. *Estimating the size of populations at risk for HIV. Issues and methods*. UNAIDS/
    IMPACT/Family Health International workshop: report and conclusions, 2002.

12 Demographic and health surveys. Available at http://www.measuredhs.com/.

13 Mercer CH, Fenton KA, Copas AJ, Wellings K, Erens B, McManus S, Nanchahal K, Macdowall W, Johnson AM. Increasing prevalence of male homosexual partnerships and practices in Britain 1990–2000: evidence from national probability surveys. *AIDS*, 2004, 18(10):1453–8.

14 Hook EB, Regal RR. Capture-recapture methods in epidemiology: methods and limitations. *Epidemiologic reviews*, 1995, 17:243–63.

15 Hickman M, Cox S, Harvey J, Howes S, Farrell M, Frischer M, Stimson G, Taylor C, Tilling K. Estimating the prevalence of problem drug use in inner London: a discussion of three capture-recapture studies. *Addiction*, 1999, 94:1653–62.

16 Platt L, Hickman M, Rhodes T, Mikhailova L, Karavashkin V, Vlasov A, Tilling K, Hope V, Khutorksoy M, Renton A. The prevalence of injecting drug use in a Russian city: implications for harm reduction and coverage. *Addiction*, 1999, 11:1430–8.

17 *European Monitoring Centre for Drugs and Drug Addiction (EMCDDA) methodological guidelines to estimate the prevalence of problem drug use on the local level.* Lisbon, EMCDDA, 1999.

Part 3

Sampling methods for HIV surveillance in community settings and in facilities

3.1

Introduction

Sampling is the selection of some individuals from a larger population to provide estimates for key measures, parameters or indicators that are reflective of the entire population [1]. Sampling consists of defining the larger or target population, developing a sampling frame or list of all persons in the population and applying a method that will select individuals from the sampling frame in an unbiased manner. When every individual in the target population has an equal or known chance of being included in the sample, the sample is held to be representative of the entire population, and measurements made on the sampled individuals (e.g. HIV seroprevalence or risk behaviour) are held to be generalizable to the entire population. Of course, the exact measure in the sample is unlikely to be precisely the figure if measured in the entire population. However, when the sample is taken so there is equal or known chance of including any particular individual, then the level of error in the sample can be calculated (e.g. "margin of error", plus or minus a few percentage points, or the 95% confidence interval). When a sample is truly representative of the population, we can be certain that comparisons between different groups within the population or comparisons between different years that the survey is repeated present a valid picture of true differences and changes in the HIV epidemic.

Ideally, the sampling frame is a list of all individuals in the population. Such a situation exists for many populations of interest to HIV surveillance, including students enrolled in a school, employees working at factories, people enlisted in the military, prisoners held in correctional facilities, and, when complete, the general population through national household-based censuses. When such complete sampling frames exist, a representative sample can be selected by assigning each individual on the list a unique number and using a random number table to pick the desired number of individuals from the list (i.e. a **simple random sample**). The approach can be modified by grouping individuals into certain geographic areas, classrooms or factories and drawing a pre-determined number randomly from each grouping (i.e. a **stratified random sample**). Simple and stratified random sampling are often done in HIV surveillance to measure HIV seroprevalence and risk behaviour for such target populations as students, teachers, workers, uniformed military personnel or prisoners and for the general population (such as in the demographic and health surveys or AIDS indicator surveys).

However, for many populations of great interest to HIV surveillance, such as most-at-risk populations, no complete lists of the entire population exist. Most-at-risk populations such as MSM, IDU and FSW are highly stigmatized and engage in what is often illegal behaviour. Household censuses are often very useful in collecting information used to monitor HIV in a given community. Unfortunately because of the hidden nature of most-at-risk populations, household censuses are unlikely to accurately record whether individuals engage in male-to-male sex, drug use or commercial sex. Moreover, if such questions are asked and answered truthfully, these populations are often so rare in the general population that it becomes exceedingly difficult and costly to meet sample size requirements. HIV surveillance must therefore create approximations of sampling frames in order to generate data that are as representative and generalizable as possible for most-at-risk populations. At present, there are several sampling approaches for most-at-risk populations commonly used in HIV surveillance that are held to produce samples that are moderately representative and reproducible over time. These include: **cluster-based sampling**, **time-location sampling** and **respondent-driven sampling**. HIV surveillance accepts that these methods may not be perfectly representative of the target population; however, the approach can be standardized and applied in a manner to be **inclusive** and **reproducible**. Inclusiveness permits assessment of different groups within the population; reproducibility permits assessment of changes in the epidemic over time.

In some circumstances, the population of interest can be found in large numbers at certain clinics, services or facilities. Such clients are enrolled as a **facility-** or **clinic-based sample** for HIV surveillance under the assumption that they are **proxies** or closely resemble the real population of interest. For example, pregnant women at antenatal clinics (ANC) are held to be proxies for the general population of sexually active women; male military personnel are held to be proxies for the general population of young men); or STI clinic patients are held to be proxies for persons with multiple sex partners (or sometimes for FSW, clients of FSW, or MSM). When the risk behaviour of the clients of these facilities is high, then they are held to be **sentinels** for HIV surveillance; that is, when HIV appears in a population it is likely to be detected first at STI clinics, drug treatment centres or prisons, for example. The term **hiv sentinel surveillance** originates from this feature. The selection of individuals in a clinic-based sample may be done by taking a random sample of clients, taking a consecutive sample of clients for a certain period or taking a systematic sample (e.g. every 10th patient). The clinics or facilities used in HIV surveillance can be selected to be inclusive of different geographic areas [2]. Moreover, if the characteristics of the clients of the facilities remain stable over time, then the samples are held to be reproducible. Under these assumptions, clinic-based samples are used to compare different populations and to track changes in the epidemic over time.

In many circumstances in HIV surveillance, a true population-based sample, an approximation of a probability-based sample or even a proxy sample is not possible. In such cases, **convenience sampling** may be the only option. Convenience sampling is when measures are taken from the most easily found individuals of the population, such as those responding to an advertisement, or online, or persons known to outreach workers. For example, **snowball sampling** is a form of convenience sampling whereby known MSM, IDU or FSW are asked to recruit as many others in the population as they can [3]. A convenience sample can be forced to be more inclusive by **purposive sampling**, whereby qualitative information from key informants guides who to include in the sample in order to obtain different perspectives [4]. When no new information is obtained with additional interviews, a point of saturation is said to be achieved. On a larger scale, **targeted sampling** uses qualitative data and estimates of the make-up of the population to guide recruitment by quotas (e.g. the proportion of women or young people to be included in a sample of IDU) [5]. However, convenience sampling cannot ensure that every member of the population has an equal or known chance of inclusion in the sample, nor that the sample is inclusive of all parts of the population, nor that it can be reproduced in the same manner from year to year to track trends. Such sampling methods are often used in the pre-surveillance assessment to provide rapid preliminary data useful for applying other sampling methods for the more developed HIV surveillance system.

A comprehensive HIV surveillance system should ultimately strive for the highest level of inclusiveness and representativeness possible that is feasible with the resources available. Unfortunately, high levels of inclusiveness, reproducibility and representativeness come at high cost. It is not possible to conduct true population-based surveys of all populations of interest in all locations on a frequent basis. This may be particularly the case in the low-level and concentrated epidemics that prevail in the Middle East and North Africa. This chapter therefore provides the rationale, assumptions and procedures for the sampling methods that are considered the most efficient at tracking the key measures of the HIV epidemic worldwide and in the region.

3.2

Sampling for HIV surveillance in community settings

HIV surveillance surveys conducted in community settings have a higher chance of obtaining inclusive and representative samples because not all members of the populations of interest attend facilities, clinics or other services. HIV surveillance that involves reaching out and recruiting members of the population of interest also fosters increased understanding of the population and the environments where they live and work. However, community-based surveys can be challenging for reasons of time, cost, complexity and safety. Moreover, since a complete list of all members of the population of interest does not exist, the sampling methods used for community-based surveillance surveys cannot guarantee complete inclusiveness and representativeness. Nonetheless, there are several sampling methods for community-based surveys that are commonly used for HIV surveillance worldwide and that are held to approximate inclusive, representative and reproducible samples. This section describes several feasible sampling methods for most-at-risk populations in HIV surveillance: cluster-based sampling, time-location sampling and respondent-driven sampling.

3.2.1 Cluster-based sampling

Ideally, a representative sample is made when the sampling frame or list contains every individual in the population of interest and a simple random sample of individuals from the list is drawn. Individuals are then contacted, and key measures are taken, such as drawing blood for HIV testing and interviews for risk behaviour. However, such a process can be very costly and time-consuming especially if the individuals are widely scattered or when establishing a list of all individuals would be challenging in itself.

To gain efficiency, **cluster-based sampling** can be done. Instead of selecting individuals, cluster-based sampling entails grouping the target population into identifiable units (e.g. towns, neighbourhoods, city blocks), numbering the groups, randomly selecting a number of groups and recruiting all individuals or a sample of individuals within the selected groups. In this manner, each member of the population has equal or known chance of inclusion; however, they are chosen as a group. The grouping that is randomly selected is referred to as the **primary sampling unit** or PSU [13]. Cluster-based sampling can be **single-stage** (where a simple random sample of groups is selected) or **multi-stage** (for example, selecting a random set of neighbourhoods in a city, followed by randomly selecting a set of streets within the neighbourhoods). In cluster-based sampling, not every group will be visited, and therefore a complete list of all individuals in the population is not required. Compared to a simple random sample of the population, the precision of cluster-based sample estimates is usually lower; that is, the margin of error is often wider depending how similar persons are to each other within the cluster.

General population surveys that employ cluster-based sampling and are widely used for public health and surveillance include the multiple indicator cluster survey (UNICEF; available at http://www.unicef.org/statistics/index_24302.html) and for HIV surveillance the demographic and health surveys and the AIDS indicator surveys (available at www.measuredhs.com). These population-based surveys are usually done at the national level and include multi-stage sampling whereby the population is divided into strata by provinces or urban and rural districts. Within these strata, villages, blocks or clusters of houses are randomly selected as PSU, followed by another stage of random selection of households. Such surveys have been used to calibrate HIV prevalence determined in ANC sentinel surveillance data for the purpose of projecting more valid estimates of HIV prevalence (see below).

HIV surveillance surveys of most-at-risk populations can be done using an approximation of cluster-based sampling when the population of interest is concentrated in certain areas or facilities whereby their numbers can be counted or estimated within the areas. For example, some at-risk populations reside or can be found in relatively fixed locations with known or estimated numbers, such as prisoners in prisons, military and police at barracks, brothel-based sex workers, lorry drivers employed at transportation companies or factory workers. In these settings, a mapping or listing of all locations can be established along with the corresponding known or estimated numbers of persons at each location. The list of locations serves as the sampling frame: a random sample of locations is selected and individuals at the randomly selected location are recruited for the survey. Sampling can be done in stages; for example, first randomly selecting prisons, then prison cell blocks, then cells, then prisoners within cells.

Of course, when the locations of interest are hidden (e.g. brothels), sampling frame development can take up a substantial amount of time. Considerable pre-surveillance and formative work is needed for cluster-based sampling of most-at-risk populations. A useful guideline for conducting this type of cluster-based sampling has been produced by Family Health International [27]: *Behavioral surveillance surveys: guidelines for repeated behavioral surveys in populations at risk for HIV*. Of note, there are several variations of cluster-based sampling and time-location sampling (TLS; see below), and their methods often overlap.

The following outlines a few common approaches to implementing cluster-based sampling for HIV surveillance in most-at-risk populations. Three phases can be defined:

- **pre-surveillance/formative assessment**, consisting of preparatory activities to identify the types and locations of sites to be included through interviews with key informants, focus groups, observation, existing programmatic data, literature review; this phase can also identify key topics to include in the preparation of the questionnaire
- **construction of a sampling frame** of all the sites or locations to be included in the survey, along with enumeration (i.e. counting) or estimation (e.g. by key informants)

Table 3.1 Selection of PSU by probability proportional to size

PSU number	Measure of size	Cumulative size	Sample selection number	Mark the PSU selected
1	120	120	72	×
2	115	235		
3	63	298		
4	92	390		
5	163	553	433.55	×
6	133	686		
7	159	845	795.1	×
⋮	⋮	⋮		
42 (last)	145	7231 (*M*)		
Total	**7231**			

Based on *Behavioral surveillance surveys. Guidelines for repeated behavioral surveys in populations at risk of HIV.* Durham, North Carolina, Family Health International, 2000.

Planned number of PSU = 20

Sampling interval = 7231/20 = 361.55

Random start between 1 and 361.55 = 72

PSU selected: 1, 5, 7.

of the numbers of individuals in the population of interest at each site (e.g. number of FSW within each brothel)

- **surveillance data collection** at the randomly selected sites, field staff approach and interview eligible respondents

For the random selection of the PSU, two basic approaches can be used: one based on the probability of inclusion proportional to the relative sizes of the PSU and one based on equal probability of inclusion of all PSU, as discussed below.

Selecting primary sampling units by probability proportional to size

The **probability proportional to size** (PPS) approach for randomly selecting PSU is used when information on the size of each PSU is relatively well known, i.e. when the number of people at each PSU is relatively stable and can be counted. In the PPS approach, larger PSU have a higher likelihood of selection for the sample than smaller PSU in direct relation to their relative sizes. This means that all individuals within all PSU have an equal probability of selection and the sample is **self-weighted**; no statistical adjustments are needed for the measures taken (of note, the margin of error still needs to be adjusted to account for how similar persons are within each cluster or PSU). The selection of the PSU by PPS can be done through a systematic sampling approach (e.g. choosing every nth PSU on the complete list of PSU) as outlined by the following steps (see also Table 3.1)[1]:

---

[1] Steps in the selection of a systematic random sample of PSU with the PPS approach are based on and explained in *Behavioral surveillance surveys. Guidelines for repeated behavioral surveys in populations at risk of HIV.* Durham, North Carolina, Family Health International, 2000, chapter 4 (page 39).

- prepare the list of all PSU with the number of people in each (that is, the count or estimate of the number of persons at the site) and the cumulative number of persons as the list continues
- calculate a cumulative measure of size M; that is, the total number of people in the whole sampling frame
- calculate the sampling interval (SI) by dividing the total cumulative measure of size M by the number of PSU to be selected a: $SI = M/a$
- select a random start (RS) number between 1 and SI using a random number table; compare this number with the cumulated measure of size column; the PSU within whose cumulated measure of size the number (RS) falls is the first PSU to be selected
- subsequent units are chosen by adding the SI to the number identified in the previous step: RS + SI, RS + 2SI, RS + 3SI, etc.
- this procedure is followed until the list has been exhausted; if the interval has been correctly calculated, the sample should end at the end of the list

The PPS approach is recommended when the number of people in each PSU is known and relatively stable. When the number is not well known or less stable, an equal probability approach may be more suitable, or a different version of sampling by sites (e.g. TLS; see below) should be used.

Selecting primary sampling units by equal probability

In the equal probability approach, each PSU has equal chance of inclusion in the random sample regardless of its size. This will lead to members of large PSU having smaller probabilities of being selected compared to members of smaller PSU. To correct for these unequal selection probabilities, data need to be weighted during the analysis (see below). Weighting requires counting or estimating the number of persons at the PSU during the pre-surveillance or formative phase or during the actual surveillance data collection phase (i.e. after the PSU have been selected). This approach works best when the number of target group members that are associated with PSU is roughly comparable; that is, when the size of each PSU does not vary greatly. An equal probability sample of PSU can be done by simple random sampling from the list of all PSU, or systematically (i.e. every nth PSU) from a random starting (RS) number (Table 3.2)[1].

Selecting individuals within a PSU

In the second stage of sampling, participants from the population of interest are chosen from the individuals found at each randomly sampled PSU or site who are determined by field staff to be eligible (e.g. member of the population of interest, age criteria, residence criteria, etc.).

When the PPS sampling approach is used, the probability of the PSU being included was based on the size of the PSU. Therefore, an equal number of individuals are recruited at each site. For example, if the total sample size needed is 400 (see below), and the number of PSU selected is 20, then 20 persons per site are enrolled in the survey. The selection of the 20 individuals can be done as a simple random sample (e.g. in a brothel containing

---

[1]   Steps in the selection of a systematic random sample of PSU with the equal probability approach is based on and explained in *Behavioral surveillance surveys. Guidelines for repeated behavioral surveys in populations at risk of HIV*. Durham, North Carolina, Family Health International, 2000, chapter 4 (page 40).

Table 3.2 Selection of PSU by equal probability approach

PSU number	Mark the PSU selected
1	
2	
3	×
4	
5	
6	
7	×
⋮	
42 (last)	
Total	

Based on *Behavioral surveillance surveys. Guidelines for repeated behavioral surveys in populations at risk of HIV.* Durham, North Carolina, Family Health International, 2000.

Planned number of PSU = 10

Sampling interval = 42/10 = 42

Random start between 1 and 42 = 3 (example).

40 rooms, number all rooms in a brothel from 1 to 40 then use a random number table to select 20 individual rooms) or systematic sampling (e.g. number all 40 rooms in the brothel, pick a random number to start at, select every second room).

When using the equal probability approach, a fixed number is also selected at each PSU (for example, 20 at 20 PSU for a sample of 400) using a simple random sample or systematic sample. However, the total number of the population present at the selected PSU needs to be counted or estimated in order to weight the data during analysis. That is, since large and small sites have equal chance of being selected, persons at small sites have higher chance of inclusion in the survey than persons at large sites. This distortion can be corrected at the analysis phase using the relative sizes of the population at the PSU.

A few additional tips and rules of thumb apply to cluster-based sampling.

- For reasonable precision of estimates (i.e. low margin of error), it is better to select more PSU and enrol a smaller number of respondents than to select fewer PSU and enrol a large number in each; for example, it is better to select 10 individuals from 40 PSU than 40 individuals from 10 PSU.
- For efficiency in the field, however, it may be wise to enrol a minimum number of participants for each PSU, for example at least 5 to 10. If individuals within the PSU share very similar characteristics or behaviour (i.e. high homogeneity), the number of respondents per PSU should be decreased, and the number of PSU increased.
- In some instances, the PSU may be small, in which case all persons present might be included, and subsequent visits may have to be made if potentially eligible persons were absent at the time of the survey.
- When the PPS approach is used, record the number of people at the site at the time of the data collection anyway. If this number is substantially different from what was found

during the initial mapping, then it may be necessary to weight the data appropriately at the analysis stage (i.e. the numbers present at the PSU were not stable).

- When doing subsequent rounds of surveys for the population, the map of PSU and the counting of persons at the PSU need to be updated. Depending on the situation, the map may retain a large proportion of PSU from year to year making subsequent construction of sampling frames less time-consuming. On the other hand, many of the specific sites may change or close or new ones appear, and formative assessment will need to keep abreast of these changes.

The forms used in selection of PSU by PPS and equal probability are in appendixes 3.4–3.6, which guide the documentation of the information to be collected for each cluster, namely:

- the procedures for defining, identifying and selecting PSU
- the list of PSU (along with any identifying information)
- the estimated size of the population at the PSU
- the number of PSU selected
- the sampling interval and random start number
- information obtained during surveillance data collection
- the cluster number and location
- the total number of people invited to participate
- the number of people who are ineligible
- the number of people who refuse to participate (list the reasons for non-participation)
- the number of duplicates or suspected duplicates
- the number of completed interviews and specimen collections.

Organization in the field: an example

The following is an example of an HIV surveillance survey using cluster-based sampling to enrol a sample of 450 sex workers. The number of sex workers per PSU is estimated to be between 10 and 20. A total of 30 PSU were chosen, and 15 women per PSU were to be enrolled. The survey coordinator planned to have two interviewers working per PSU and three field teams total. Assuming it will take one team a day to interview 15 women (i.e. that one interviewer can interview seven women per day), then one team can complete five PSU per week, and 15 PSU can be done by three teams in a week (see Table 3.3). However, difficulties encountered in the field (i.e. respondents not present at the site when interviewers are there, interviewing proceeding more slowly than planned, or sites might be distant from one another) may lengthen the time to complete the sample. For such reasons, the number of PSU to be sampled should be increased by, for example, 10%, in this case selecting 33 instead of 30.

Table 3.3 Cluster-based sampling: calculation of time to completion of sample

	One team	Three teams
Daily	15 women (1 PSU)	45 women (3 PSU)
Weekly	75 women (5 PSU)	225 women (15 PSU)
Two weeks	150 women (10 PSU)	450 women (30 PSU)

3.2.2 Time-location sampling

Time-location sampling (TLS) is a version of cluster-based sampling used when the population of interest is mobile and variable in numbers at the gathering sites or venues. TLS has been widely used for bio-behavioural HIV surveillance surveys and has been described in the literature [15, 16, 17]. Further details on the rationale, methods and analysis of TLS data can be found in *Resource guide: time-location sampling (TLS)* accessible at http://globalhealthsciences.ucsf.edu/PPHG/surveillance/resources.html.

Groups that can be sampled by TLS include street-based FSW, MSM at bars and cruising areas, lorry drivers at stops at cross-roads or along corridors of transportation and IDU in shooting galleries and other public venues. The condition for TLS is that target groups gather or concentrate at certain sites or venues during specific times of day and days of the week. For example, there might be more FSW at certain bus stops or street corners during the weekend or MSM at bars on certain nights of the week. In TLS, the PSU is defined as the venue and the day of the week and the time period of the day (i.e. the VDT). Thus, the same site may have more than one VDT available for scheduling sampling events. A difference from cluster-based sampling is that the number of the target population at the PSU is highly variable and there is uncertainty that the number counted during the formative phase will be the same as when conducting recruitment and data collection.

In TLS, a comprehensive map or list of all VDT is constructed as the sampling frame. TLS starts with identifying the universe of all venues and the days, times, and characteristics of people in attendance. Mapping is both physical and ethnographic and is accomplished through key informant interviews of population members and other gatekeepers, focus group discussions, examination of existing information and observation in the field through visiting the potential gathering places. Approval for visiting and sampling venues should be sought from owners of these venues during preparations for the survey. TLS allows for the addition of further venues to the sampling frame during data collection. TLS depends heavily on knowledge of the diversity of venues where the population of interest can be found and is therefore most successful when well informed community guides and members of the target population are included in all stages. Because the target population will circulate through venues, success in the field for TLS also depends on having a single field leader and low staff turn-over to remember faces to limit duplication.

TLS is appropriate for populations who are not fixed in a venue but rather move freely about and to other venues. These populations may include:

- young people out of school—markets, parks, bus stations, street corners
- female sex workers—street corners, bars, hotels
- men who have sex with men—bars, cruising areas, dance clubs
- injection drug users—shooting galleries, street corners
- lorry drivers—lorry stops, customs posts.

During the early stages of creating the sampling frame, a rapid count (i.e. enumeration) and brief interview are conducted to assess if the persons present would be eligible (i.e. members of the target group). If attendance varies according to time and the subpopulation present, then the week should be divided into days and days into time intervals according to the variations in attendance pattern and type. The PSU comprise the distinct venue, day and time periods and are entered separately into the listing of PSU for the sampling frame.

Since the relative numbers of the population are fluid, the PSU are usually selected by the equal probability approach described for cluster-based sampling above. Recruitment and data collection usually take place for a fixed time interval for each sampling event at the selected PSU. For example, a four-hour period for recruitment usually allows for one complete staff shift with time for set-up, transportation and debriefing, while at the same time the population present at the venue will be relatively stable with a short enough interval to avoid duplication.

Basic steps for TLS

- Create a map and list all the sites or venues where members of most-at-risk populations congregate established through formative assessment.
- Based on the results from mapping, decide criteria to be included in the sampling frame: each site can be included in the sampling frame once with its corresponding high attendance daytime periods (e.g. minimum numbers present to qualify for inclusion). One site can be included, for example, as one weekday night, one weekend afternoon and one weekend evening.
- Collect information on the approximate number of target group members that attend sites during the specific time periods (i.e. during mapping) and basic sociodemographic and behavioural profiles. Sites should be included only at times when target group members congregate, preferably at the busiest times.
- Decide on the sample size (see below) and, using a minimum efficiency factor (e.g. minimum of eight surveys completed per sampling event), determine how many sampling events will be needed to reach the sample size.
- Scheduling recruitment events is best if done in one-month increments. A month of sampling events selected at random gives adequate opportunity for a number of venues to be randomly selected and reduces potential burden on any one venue (e.g. if randomly selecting a week of events at a time random chance could dictate that one particular venue is drawn each week, thus increasing the burden on that venue and decreasing variability in the range of venues sampled). For each month from the set of available venues (PSU) use simple random sampling to select the needed number of venues to meet the needed number of sampling events. Furthermore, using PSU with similar daytime periods, randomly selected alternates can be scheduled to ensure that valuable staff time will not be lost if the primary venue is unexpectedly not busy, closed or unavailable due to external factors. In addition, one-time events (e.g. a special NGO mobilization event) may be purposefully added to the sampling frame in limited numbers.
- Sampling should take the same amount of time at each site (e.g. four hours).
- At each sampling event, the field leader counts all present at the VDT during the entire sampling period (i.e. a complete count of all the target population present is made, regardless of whether they complete the survey). These data are needed for weighting data during analysis. Of note, one field leader conducts the enumeration and designates field staff to intercept and interview potentially eligible persons.
- At each sampling event, population members are systematically sampled (e.g. every fifth person) or consecutively included (i.e. every person until all staff are occupied) by the field leader without staff choice. In practice, recruitment (but not counting) is suspended when all staff are interviewing participants. Once staff are again available, recruitment resumes.

- A set number of surveys completed at each sampling event is not required, although some versions of TLS do target a fixed number per recruitment event. For efficiency, recruitment may continue until the end of the sampling event (e.g. the predetermined four-hour period). Should recruitment be slow and it seems minimum goals for interviews may not be met, surveillance teams may consider going to the randomly selected alternate venue.

Attention must be paid not to sample the same individuals who move across different sites. This presents a challenge to TLS. Avoiding duplication may best be accomplished through having a single field leader and a consistent recruitment team to recognize individuals. In addition, the initial intercept to assess eligibility should be clear that persons cannot participate more than once. Other techniques include "biometrics" such as wrist circumference and routine examination of surveys with similar data (e.g. date of birth, education level and other demographic factors).

As in conventional cluster-based sampling, in TLS it is crucial to document the PSU selection process and the selection within each PSU. In particular, this includes recording:

- the number of people appearing at the site during the entire observation period
- the number of people asked to participate in the survey
- the number of people eligible for the survey
- the number of completed interviews and blood draws
- the number of refusals (and if possible reasons why)
- the number of duplicates or potential duplicates.

Further detail of the basic steps of TLS are provided below.

Formative assessment and enumeration

The aim of the formative assessment and enumeration is to determine if venues and their associated time periods are attended by sufficient numbers of potential participants to be included in the sampling frame. Enumeration is done as part of mapping in TLS in two phases: type 1 enumeration consists of counting only people at the site who are roughly presumed all to be target group members but *not* counting people who are obviously not members of the priority group. (i.e. as a rapid assessment of the venue), and type 2 enumeration consists of counting and a brief interview to assess eligibility for definitive inclusion in the sampling frame.

Type 1 enumeration

At each potential venue identified through key informants, focus groups and other sources, an enumerator counts the number of persons who appear at the site and may meet the inclusion criteria and who enter a defined enumeration area or cross an enumeration line for the first time during a 30–60 minute period. For example, for MSM the enumerator would count adult men who are entering a gay bar or are hanging out in a cruising area. Area- or line-based enumeration may be conducted depending on the physical environment of the venue and constraints for space during the surveillance data collection; for either method, enumeration should be conducted outside but near the venue entrance.

- **Area-based enumeration** defines a zone which potentially eligible persons enter. Area-based enumeration should be conducted at sites such as street corners, parks, bars and dance clubs. All persons entering the area may be recruited (during the data collection phase) and only those who enter the area for the first time are counted.
- **Line-based enumeration** defines a line which potentially eligible persons cross, such as a section of a street. Line-based enumeration should be conducted at venues with a high flow of target group members. People entering or leaving the venue are enumerated as they cross an imaginary line placed near the venue entrance.

Once the area or line is defined, for 30 to 60 minutes the enumerator counts people who appear to meet the inclusion criteria who enter or cross it. Only persons who cross the line for the first time are counted. After enumerations are conducted, counts are standardized to a two- or four-hour period, which is assumed to be the minimum (or in some cases average) duration of a sampling event. For example, if 5 men were counted in a 30-minute (0.5 hours) period entering a gay bar, then the standardized count for a full four-hour recruitment event would be 40 (= 5/0.5 × 4). The standardized counts allow for judging whether the VDT should be included in the sampling frame (e.g. a large enough number of eligible men) and for planning the number of recruitment events needed. For example, the decision could be made to only include VDT where a minimum of 10 persons would be recruited in a four-hour period.

For many venues, the type 1 enumeration may be very brief. For example, simple visual inspection may rapidly determine that ample numbers are present at the venue, or that the venue is closed, has moved or too few persons are in attendance. For some venues, it may take more information to determine if a sufficient number of the target population is truly present, requiring a type 2 enumeration.

Type 2 enumeration

The purpose of type 2 enumeration is to ensure correct inclusion of venues and daytime periods where it is not clear if a high proportion of attendees are members of the target population and to better understand the characteristics of people who attend the sites, including age, sex and most-at-risk population membership. Type 2 enumerations should be considered for those venues where the demographic and risk characteristics are not obvious through a rapid assessment or venues that might not include sufficient numbers of eligible subjects. As in the type 1 enumeration, one staff member counts people who enter an enumeration area or pass an enumeration line during a 30–60 minute period and generates an expected yield while another staff member performs brief interviews with a consecutive sample of those counted. Counting and consecutive interviewing is performed for 30–60 minutes, and then standardized to two- or four-hour periods. "Consecutive interviews" does not imply that every person counted is approached. It means that people are approached as staff are available. During interviews, a form records data on a person's key characteristics (e.g. age, race/ethnicity, type of drug use). The brief interview questions should address the inclusion criteria, such as age, sexual orientation, or drug use; however, this type of enumeration is not the surveillance data collection itself. Rather, it is to ensure proper inclusion of venues in the sampling frame.

Random selection of venues and associated daytime periods

Once the universe of venues (i.e. sampling frame) is complete, surveillance teams prepare for sampling. To construct a sampling calendar (workplan), a two-stage random selection is conducted. First venues are randomly selected from the universe of venues. This is done without replacement, meaning that once selected for the month's calendar they are not put back in the sampling frame. Then from each venue's list of daytime periods one daytime period is randomly selected and scheduled on the surveillance team's sampling calendar. In addition an alternate venue can be randomly selected for each primary venue. Alternate venues ensure teams will be able to effectively use their time for data collection should primary venues be unavailable on a particular randomly selected day and time. Details of creating a sampling calendar can be found at http://globalhealthsciences.ucsf. edu/PPHG/surveillance/resources.html: *Time-location sampling resource guide.*

Selecting and enrolling participants in TLS

In the data collection stage of the survey, recruitment of individuals at each randomly selected venue is systematic (e.g. every or every *n*th person as long as staff are available). The field team leader (who is enumerating all persons entering the area) designates staff to intercept target group members who cross a designated line or enter a designated area to be approached for screening questions. If more than one person is entering the designated area, a staff member can approach the one that is the closest. Staff can be scattered evenly throughout the site area to be able to encounter people who come from different directions. The key element in approaching potential participants is to minimize any selectivity on the part of data collection staff. Staff should approach each potential participant as they are ready.

The designated person is approached, and the study is briefly introduced. If the intercepted person agrees to a few screening questions, they are assessed for eligibility. If eligible, then full informed consent is performed in a private area nearby or in a van parked near the venue. After consent, the interview is conducted, pre-test counselling is performed, and blood is drawn for HIV and STI testing. At the end of the data and specimen collection, appropriate counselling and referral for needed services are made. In addition, an appointment is made for results disclosure and post-test counselling.

Performance criteria

Performance criteria are set before sampling begins to provide data collection teams with a way to monitor their progress, ensure sample size is met in the data collection period, maintain high quality data and to ensure maximum participation and efficiency. Performance should be adapted for each study and monitored for each event, and feedback given to the field team.

Typical performance criteria to achieve a rigorous sample for a survey of a most-at-risk population with a sample size of 500:

- data collection for no less than one month and no more than three months
- completing at least 14 sampling events per month
- a minimum of 8–12 completed interviews per event
- completing 100% of sampling events

- complete ≥ 90% of the intercepts
- enrol ≥ 75% of the eligible men
- collect specimens with 80% of enrolled men
- 500 subjects total.

Weights and analysis of TLS data

TLS is held to approximate random sampling in that each venue/VDT has an equal chance of inclusion. Given a high chance that individuals in target populations will attend an included venue and if enough venues/VDTs sampled, with no bias in selection of venue/VDT or selection of subjects, TLS approximates a random sampling of the population. Nonetheless, differences in attendance patterns and differences in who attends certain venues does potentially introduce different sampling probabilities and clustering of similar people at venues.

Several different weighting methods and statistical adjustments have been proposed for TLS, and methods are still under development. However, in practice weighting has not often been used because key outcomes were not found to be associated with venues and venues have shown high heterogeneity of attendees. Moreover, TLS usually produces many small clusters rather than a few large homogenous clusters which generally tends to minimize design effects and changes between crude and adjusted analyses. Nonetheless, it may be necessary to statistically adjust data collected using TLS. This will particularly be the case when a small number of large clusters makes up the survey sample.

We present here a simplified approach based on enumeration counts of each sampling event which produce probability weights (p weights). Weighting can be achieved by using the enumeration count of each event as the basis for the weight.

In brief, the adjustment should produce estimates that reflect the ratio of the number of persons enrolled to the number of eligible persons at each recruitment event. If the same ratio is conserved across all recruitment events then the sample is self-weighted and no adjustment would be needed.

To show how to weight, the following table (Table 3.4) illustrates a fictional TLS study, the enumeration counts for each event and the total number of interviews completed at each of those events. Column 2 shows the total number of potential subjects enumerated at each event, column 3 is the proportion that each event represents of the total enumeration count for the entire study (for event 2 that would be 107/6678 = 0.016023), column 4 is the total number of interviews completed at each event and column 5 is the proportion of the total number of completed interviews that each event represents (for event 2 that is 19/435 = 0.043678). Finally column 6 shows the calculated p weight for each event (for event 2, 0.016023/0.043678 = 0.366836904). This p weight would then be applied to each interview completed during that event.

Table 3.4 Weighting example

1	2	3	4	5	6
Event ID	Enumeration count	p of enumeration	Interview count	p of interview	p weight
1	16	0.002396	1	0.002299	1.042228212
2	107	0.016023	19	0.043678	0.366836904
3	67	0.010033	11	0.025287	0.396757331
4	60	0.008985	10	0.022989	0.39083558
5	913	0.136718	20	0.045977	2.973607367
6	353	0.05286	15	0.034483	1.532943995
7	102	0.015274	22	0.050575	0.302009311
8	65	0.009733	10	0.022989	0.423405211
9	132	0.019766	23	0.052874	0.373842728
10	397	0.059449	19	0.043678	1.361067764
11	443	0.066337	22	0.050575	1.311667892
12	235	0.03519	25	0.057471	0.612309075
13	195	0.0292	24	0.055172	0.529256514
14	189	0.028302	23	0.052874	0.535274815
15	3	0.000449	3	0.006897	0.065139263
16	59	0.008835	6	0.013793	0.640536089
17	100	0.014975	14	0.032184	0.465280452
18	470	0.07038	27	0.062069	1.133905694
19	181	0.027104	17	0.03908	0.693541568
20	654	0.097934	21	0.048276	2.02862277
21	85	0.012728	8	0.018391	0.692104672
22	509	0.07622	20	0.045977	1.65779425
23	190	0.028452	20	0.045977	0.618823001
24	88	0.013178	6	0.013793	0.955375861
25	89	0.013327	7	0.016092	0.828199204
26	409	0.061246	18	0.041379	1.480108815
27	217	0.032495	17	0.03908	0.831483537
28	350	0.05241l	7	0.016092	3.256963163
Totals	6678	1	435	1	27.49992104

Enumeration counts for each event must be attached to each observation made at that event. There are two main ways to accomplish this. If using paper and pencil instruments, the enumeration count for each event can be recorded on the cover of each survey completed at that event. Enumeration counts for each event can be added to each observation in your final dataset after data collection has ended. Thus, simple fractions for groups of participants are based on the relative numbers of persons at the venues when recruitment occurred.

Adjustment for clustering

In the case where venues do attract similar types of people, there may be substantial homogeneity among persons sampled at each venue. This homogeneity can result in a widening of the standard errors of estimates (i.e. the margin of error). Standard errors need to be adjusted accordingly using standardized commands in statistical software packages (e.g. Sudaan, SAS or in survey commands in Stata). Statistical software provides these adjustments by designating the venue as the group or cluster. Again, in typical practice where the number of venues is high, the number of subjects per venue is small and there is heterogeneity at the venue, the adjustments to the standard errors will likely be small.

Should your formative assessment or field experience indicate that a venue is differently attended by very different members of the most-at-risk population during specific daytime periods, then each period could be counted as a separate cluster. In practice, this distinction should already have been addressed by adding these venues to the universe of venues as separate unique venues with their own unique VDT.

Effect of weighting and cluster analysis: an example

To show how the weighting may change the point estimates and standard errors in a TLS study, an example adapted from a real-life survey of MSM in San Francisco (n = 435) is presented. The crude data, which are treated as a simple random sample, show the proportion reporting any unprotected receptive anal intercourse as 24.49 % (standard error [SE] 2.38). Standard errors, produced by statistical analyses when analysing sample data, are necessary to calculate confidence intervals.

Adjustment using the survey weights based on attendance and sampling fractions as described above produces the proportion practising unprotected receptive anal intercourse as 25.7912% (SE 2.5677).

Accounting for the clustering effect of each venue-day-time sampling event, that is taking into account the homogeneity of persons attending a specific venue (34 in this case), the adjustment produces a proportion practising unprotected receptive anal intercourse as 24.4898% (SE 2.6127).

Combining both the weighting and clustering adjustment estimates the proportion as 25.7912% (SE 2.721).

Comparing the crude estimates to the adjusted finds a small relative change in the point estimate (about 5% of the overall point estimate), whereas there is a nearly 17% change in the standard error. Such changes suggest that in this survey point estimates may not change too severely; however, interpretation of differences and odds ratios predicting unprotected receptive anal intercourse may change when the sample is weighted.

Staffing for TLS

- A **field team** needs to be established for each of the priority groups to be surveyed. It is desirable to have members of the priority population be members of the field team for multiple reasons, including to assist with venue identification and characterization, eligibility assessment, questionnaire development (in language and terms familiar to the population), recruitment and interviewing. Field teams consist of a minimum of three persons (two interviewers and field coordinator), with more interviewers added as needed.
- A **study coordinator** or **study supervisor** implements the protocol, ensures adherence to procedures and monitors data collection. The study coordinator may be the same as the field coordinator depending on the scope of the surveys.
- A **field coordinator** leads the team in identifying clusters to be included in the sampling frame (venues for TLS), distinguishing individual PSU (VDT for TLS) and the approximate number of people within each PSU. The field coordinator accompanies the recruitment teams in the field and directs intercept of individuals for approach and recruitment.
- **Interviewers** administer the questionnaire and collect biological specimens (some locations require staff to be clinically trained to collect specimens). All need to receive training in interviewing techniques and the protection of confidentiality and participants' rights. It is highly desirable that interviewers be members of the most-at-risk population among which surveillance is being conducted.
- In studies where physical examinations, collection of biological specimens, HIV counselling or STI treatment is done, a **medically trained person** (physician, nurse) may be required on the team.
- When serological or other testing is conducted, a **laboratory technician** is also designated for the team. The technician ensures appropriate specimen collection, materials, labelling, handling and transport to the laboratory as well as the quality assurance in the laboratory.

3.2.3 Respondent-driven sampling

In many situations, the population of interest is hidden, may not concentrate in particular visible locations or cannot be directly approached by surveillance staff and researchers. This may be the case for MSM in settings where male–male sex is illegal and for IDU and FSW when police sweeps are frequent. Such settings make cluster-based and TLS sampling approaches difficult. An option for sampling most-at-risk populations called respondent-driven sampling (RDS) addresses many of these challenges [18, 19, 20]. The detailed description of RDS methods and procedures is based on the following source: Johnston LG. *Conducting respondent driven sampling (RDS) studies in diverse settings: a training manual for planning RDS studies.* Atlanta, Georgia, Centers for Disease Control and Prevention, 2007. The following section describes the underlying principles and basic steps of RDS.

RDS is a variant of a long chain-referral method for recruitment that does not require the development of a sampling frame of individuals or mapping of the universe of venues where the target population can be found. In practice, RDS resembles "snowball" sampling whereby members of the population recruit other members of the population within their social networks. However, unlike snowball sampling, recruitment is done in a controlled manner while collecting data that can be used to adjust for the biases entailed in persons recruiting from their social networks. RDS is based on the theory that high-risk groups within geographic areas are more or less completely linked through social networks, that they can identify and find one another and, if chains of recruitment progress long enough, then the data collected can be used to produce population estimates.

RDS starts with the selection of a limited number of initial respondents (seeds) who are non-randomly selected from the target population. The seeds are asked to recruit into the study a limited number of other members of the target population (typically three), and their recruits are similarly asked to recruit others, and so on, forming a series of "waves". When referral chains progress long enough (typically four to six waves), subsequent waves are independent of the starting seeds and the sample composition stabilizes or reaches "equilibrium" [20, 23]. At equilibrium, the data can be weighted to approximate probability sampling using information collected on the personal network size from each respondent and tracking who recruits whom through the use of a distinctive coupon with a coding system.

It has been asserted that RDS requires less formative research than cluster-based sampling or TLS; however, a number of activities still need to be carried out as part of formative assessment. These include establishing collaboration with nongovernmental organizations and target group members, interviews with group members to explore their interest in participating, the nature of the social networks and how willing the population may be to recruiting each other, the amount of incentive required and the approximate sizes of social networks. The formative stage also identifies appropriate initial seeds to start recruitment chains. Members of the high-risk population and organizations that work with them are key partners in conducting such studies and should be included in preparations for RDS from the very beginning. For example, an NGO that works with MSM can be valuable in recruitment of seeds. Seeds are the first persons in the target group to be contacted who participate in the study and therefore are essential advocates for success in reaching others in the population. Once they complete all parts of the study they will be given an incentive (i.e. a primary incentive) for participation and up to a set number of coupons for recruitment of additional peers for the study (typically three coupons but sometimes four or five). Recruiters are given an additional incentive (i.e. a secondary incentive) for each recruit who completes the interview. The most appropriate seeds are those from the diverse subgroups of the population, those who have large social networks and those who are trusted or gatekeepers to the wider population.

RDS has several unique features. Unlike other sampling approaches, RDS does not require a sampling frame or list of all individuals in a population or a map of all venues where the population can be found. RDS reaches persons through their networks, and therefore does not require that they frequent specific venues to be included. RDS does not impose on persons who may not wish to be approached by staff at venues. RDS also masks refusal from the recruiter. The long chains of recruitment mean that RDS can reach a diverse sample of the population, with deep penetration into the network structure. Finally, in order to analyse RDS data, specialized software (at present, RDSAT) is needed to make the adjustments for recruitment patterns and network sizes.

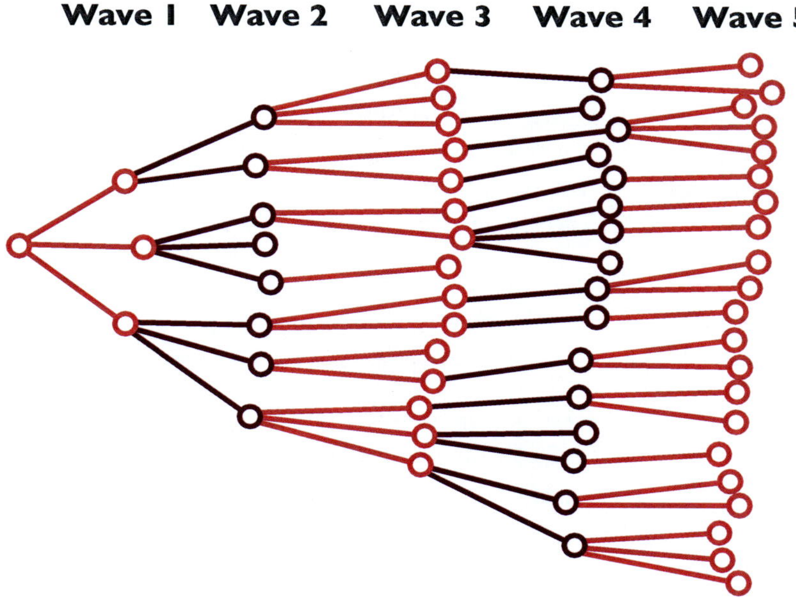

Description of the RDS process and procedures are based on the following source: Johnston LG. *Conducting respondent driven sampling (RDS) studies in diverse settings: a training manual for planning RDS studies.* Atlanta, Georgia, Centers for Disease Control and Prevention, 2007.

Figure 3.1 One seed and five waves in an example of an RDS study

Example of RDS recruitment

Let us take an example of how an RDS survey progresses. If we select 10 seeds (wave 0), and if each of them successfully refers two peers to the study, there will be 20 participants in wave 1. In wave 2, if these 20 respondents select 2 each, there will be 40. In wave 3, if these 40 select 2 each, there will be 80 respondents in wave 3. By this manner of recruitment, we can get 20 + 40 + 80 = 140 respondents (not counting seeds) by the third wave in theory. In practice, not all persons successfully recruit their peers. Generally, around 40% of possible recruitments are ultimately successful. Moreover, different chains proceed at different paces and to different lengths.

Theoretically, a sample size of 400 can be reached after four to six waves, which should be also the time when equilibrium is reached, i.e. the point at which the sample composition no longer changes. In practice, at least one or a few very long chains are usually needed since some chains will not grow. Sampling usually ends when a minimum target sample size has been reached *and* the sample has reached equilibrium. It is important to monitor the progression of recruitment as sampling progresses in order to decide when to reduce the number of coupons given per recruiter to end the sample. Conversely, the number of coupons per recruiter can be increased if recruitment lags behind target.

Formative research steps for RDS

RDS begins with a focused formative research or assessment phase. Several key issues need to be assessed to determine whether RDS can be used in the population (i.e. the population is networked) and how best to implement the study in the field; these include network size, network density, level of incentives and selection of seeds [24].

Network size

RDS can be conducted only within target populations who form social networks. In the formative phase, key informants should be asked to describe the typical size and structure of the networks in the population. Ultimately, the data collection needs to quantify as precisely as possible the size of the network for each individual—information essential to the adjusted analysis. For example, the questions may be phrased as follows.

> How many people do you know (who also know you) by name (and they know yours) who are [*target group members*]; and you have seen them in the past six months [*or past three months, or past month*]; and they live in this city/area; and you might find them again in the next two weeks?

Clearly, this question is complex and very specific to the population being sampled. For simplicity, the question may be broken up into discrete sections, recording network size for each part. Given the great importance that the network size has on the analysis of RDS data, the best way to ask this question is an area that is still under development. The formative assessment period helps determine the most appropriate way to ask this question in the specific location.

Target group members should know at least three peers who would be eligible to participate and who can be reached in a short period of time. Therefore, larger peer networks are more predictive of success of RDS in a population. For example, knowing 20 other group members for a given time period in a given area as is an indication that the target population has fairly large network sizes and may be suitable for RDS. Probing how many target group members they have met in the past month, three months and six months will help to formulate the network questions which will be used during data collection and for data analysis. The appropriate time period to assess potential network recruits is a time that will produce a network size of between 10 and 20 individuals[1]. Smaller network sizes may indicate that the population is too small or isolated for RDS; too large and quantifying the network size becomes imprecise.

Network density

Having large network sizes is an indication of the density of a target population's social networks. Density of networks refers to levels and types of social interaction. Dense networks are good for RDS as they suggest that target group members socialize together. Questions to assess density of networks are as follows.

> Could you tell me about how your peers interact with each other? (What kinds of activities do they do together?)

> Do you know [*target group members*] in [*city or province location where sites will be located*]? How often do you see them and why?

Level of incentives

Incentives should be set low enough to be non-coercive; that is they do not bring to bear undue influence that may make someone participate in the project when they may have ambivalence about participation, but high enough to cover the costs of participation and

---

[1] Having very large network sizes will not substantially affect data analysis. However, it may be easier to manage data with reasonably sized networks.

provide some motivation to participate and recruit others across different types of network. The level of incentives will vary across population groups, countries and according to local ethical standards. These ethical standards are typically available through local institutional review boards. The formative phase should determine the appropriate amount of incentive after consultation with the target population, gatekeepers, ethical boards and other researchers working with the population. In some locations, the cost of round-trip transportation from the city centre to the project site serves as a basis for estimating the correct incentive. Non-cash incentives (e.g. bus tokens, food vouchers) should also be explored.

Selection of seeds

The formative assessment is also an opportunity to identify seeds. The correct number of seeds depends on the structure of the network. Although long chain recruitment is expected and required to cross between different types of network, recruitment progresses faster if seeds are launched in distinct subnetworks (e.g. having young and old seeds, by neighbourhood, by sex). While each subnetwork should have a seed, typically 8 to 10 seeds are initially planted. Additional seeds can also be included after data collection has started if recruitment goes more slowly than planned. The best seeds are those members of the target population who are well connected (i.e. have large network sizes) to other members of the target population, well liked, respected and enthusiastically support the survey. Seeds need to be carefully instructed in the objectives and methods of survey, in techniques to recruit successfully and in how to explain recruitment to their peers. Because seeds are non-randomly selected (and they are automatically excluded by the RDS analysis software from the final analysis because of their non-randomness), they may be selected from NGO, outreach programmes or through contacts made by peer educators.

Field steps for RDS

The following list the steps for preparation and implementation of an RDS survey; further detail is provided below.

1. Determine whether RDS is suited to the target group and setting.
2. Get agreement of the key stakeholders on the appropriateness of RDS methods.
3. Establish collaboration with NGO who work with a target group.
4. Decide on HIV and STI tests, collaborating laboratory and purchase of tests.
5. Select the field site for interviewing and testing; this should be accessible and safe for the target population.
6. Select seeds.
7. Develop a questionnaire.
8. Prepare and translate all data collection forms, prepare coupon management file.
9. Prepare the application for the research ethics committee.
10. Design coupons.
11. Select staff.
12. Train staff on RDS methods, designate staff responsibilities.
13. Decide on the levels of primary and secondary incentives.
14. Design database for entering questionnaire data.
15. Transfer data into RDSAT, conduct data analysis.
16. Write report and disseminate findings and recommendations.

Steps 1–4

These activities comprise parts of the pre-assessment phase and have activities in common with other types of surveillance survey addressed in other parts of this guide. As mentioned earlier, RDS is feasible when the target population has a sufficiently dense network, is willing to visit the study site and when group members can recruit each other. The formative phase explores the appropriate level of incentives. During preparations, interviews with target group members and focus group discussions should help find information about their network size and interest in participating.

Step 5.   Select the site for interviewing and testing

Interview sites should be accessible to the population and located in an area where participants and staff feel safe. Study sites may be VCT centres, premises or storefronts of NGO that work with most-at-risk populations and health care centres. Sites used by NGO have several advantages in that staff are familiar with the target population and have interviewing skills and other resources. In some settings, the site of interview may be selected by the participant (e.g. park, gay bar, other familiar venue).

Depending on the sample size, the availability of interview sites and the geographic size of the study area, more than one site may be selected for interviewing. This requires a much stricter management of coupons and field logistics to maintain consistency and prevent duplication of participants. To manage multiple sites, study supervisors should meet preferably every day with the site managers to ensure the coupon identification numbers are not duplicated and troubleshoot issues in quality control.

The site for interviewing and testing have the following set up and flow (depending on the availability of rooms and the survey logistics and organization):

- a reception area where potential participants are screened for eligibility and informed consent is performed
- a private room for interviewing or administering of a questionnaire and pre-test counselling
- a room for blood and other biological specimen collection
- a room for the coupon manager
- money for incentives.

The times for the site to be open should be determined during the formative phase, with particular input from the target population. The hours of operation also need to be projected to accommodate the full sample size in the targeted time period. However, it might happen that recruitment goes more slowly than predicted and that the data collection period has to be extended. The site should be open for an additional two weeks to allow those that still have coupons to come, as well as those who are coming to pick up the results of laboratory tests. The interview site must remain safe and private, and all information must remain confidential.

Step 6.   Selection of seeds

As described above, selection of appropriate seeds is essential for successful chains of recruitment. Experience indicates that between 8 and 10 seeds is ideal, but depends on the structure of the networks. It is important that seeds have large social networks and are well connected with the peer group. Seeds should be diverse in respect to demographic and key variables, such as HIV status, sexual identity, drug preference, type of sex work and socioeconomic status.

Step 7. Develop a questionnaire

This phase is similar to other sampling methods except that the questionnaire for RDS includes specific questions about the network size (see above). In addition, RDS includes questions on how the recruits knew their recruiters.

Step 8. Prepare and translate all data collection forms and prepare a coupon management file

There are several forms that are used in RDS; examples are provided in appendixes 3.7–3.12.

● *Client checklist form*
This form is used to record all steps that a participant has gone through in RDS. It is completed by the staff at the site and should be designed according to the types of data collected during a survey.

● *Informed consent*
As in other surveys, informed consent explains to participants the aims of the survey, what is expected from them and the risks and benefits of participation. It needs to be either signed by a participant or agreed to orally. Oral consent is preferable to signed consent when collecting information from vulnerable groups when their signature would constitute their only connection to the study.

● *Size of the network form (essential for the RDS analysis)*
The size of the network form is best completed in the face-to-face interview before or after a participant completes a questionnaire. It asks how many target group members one knows and has seen during the specific time period (past month or past three months), and how many of them meet the inclusion criteria for a survey (see above for example). The question is essential to the statistical adjustment of the measures of the survey. The following question on the relationship between the recruiter and recruit is also needed to ensure that sampling is occurring along true social networks.

> The person who recruited you to the study is a: a) stranger, b) partner, c) family member, d) acquaintance, e) friend.

If this information indicates that most of the participants have been recruited by strangers, then the process of recruitment did not occur from the social network of the recruiter and therefore violates an underlying assumption of RDS.

● *Non-eligibility form*
The non-eligibility form is used to record those who have come to the survey site to participate but do not meet the inclusion criteria, noting which criteria have not been met.

● *Refusal forms*
Refusal forms serve to record why potential respondents refused to participate in a survey

once they had been included; reasons include fear of participation, not willing to give blood, not willing to answer certain questions in a questionnaire.

● *Coupon management file*
The coupon management file is used for data analysis. It serves to track how coupons are being distributed. This database enables tracking of the recruitment process, finding out how many recruiters have been included in the study per seed and how many valid coupons remain in circulation.

● *Coupon rejecters form (non-response form)*
The coupon rejecters form (non-response form) is completed when those who participated in the survey come to pick up secondary incentives. It is used to estimate how many of those approached refused to take coupons, what were the reasons for refusing to participate and what their basic demographic and risk profiles were (the profile of non-responders helps assess potential biases and their effects on key measures, such as HIV prevalence).

● *Financial reporting form*
The financial reporting form is used to track how much money is being spent on primary and secondary incentives for each participant and for the whole survey.

Step 9.   Prepare the application for the research ethical committee

Also common to the other types of survey, the approval of the local ethics committee is required before implementation. The application form depends on the country-specific regulations, and it is worth knowing well in advance how and when it needs to be submitted.

Step 10.   Designing coupons

The coupon is an essential part of RDS in that it links the recruit to his or her recruiter through a coding system—a necessary step for analysis. Possession of a valid coupon is an eligibility criterion for the survey. The coupon also provides clear information about the study (e.g. location of project site) and should not be easily forged. Coupons must contain a space for a **unique identification number** so that each coupon can easily link recruiters with recruits. In summary, the purpose of coupons in RDS is to:

● provide information about the study, e.g. the time and location of the study site, to potential recruits
● link information about recruits and their recruiters through the coupon numbering system
● track overall progress of recruitment and manage incentive payments to recruiters.

RDS coupons contain the following items:

● unique identification number of the participant
● unique identification number of their recruiter
● organization name
● address of interview site
● telephone number (if available)
● days and hours of site operation
● expiration date.

Each coupon has two parts that can be easily separated.

The upper part of the coupon serves as the referral coupon that the recruiter uses to recruit a peer. In the example of the coupon provided from the RDS study among MSM in Croatia, it is red (Figures 3.2 and 3.3).

The lower part of the coupon serves as the payment coupon. It is kept by the recruiter, who will use it to claim an incentive for having recruited a peer. In the example of the coupon provided from the RDS study among MSM in Croatia, it is grey (Figures 3.2 and 3.3).

Both parts of the coupon have a unique identification number for the recruit.

To reduce the possibility of the coupon duplication, an official stamp can be added over the perforation. When the upper and lower parts of the coupon are separated, one half of the stamp is on each part of the coupon.

Coupons are usually of the size of two credit cards, one placed above the other (approximately 8.5 × 10 cm).

If more than one RDS study is going on at the same time, it is best that coupons use different colours and are distinct from one another in design.

The following figures are samples of the coupons which might be used in RDS studies, though the coupon design will depend on the types of information that are relevant for a local RDS study and the target groups.

Upper front of the coupon

The top front portion is a referral coupon and contains information for the participant's recruits (shown in Figure 3.2 below in red). It includes the following information:

- the unique identification number of the recruit
- the title of the implementing organization
- a phone number, if available, and the location and address of the interview site
- the hours and days when participants can come to the site
- space for project staff to write in dates of validation of a coupon (activation and expiration date). Some projects may need to adjust this timeframe according to speed of recruitment; if recruitment goes slowly, the expiration date could be extended. It is very important that coupons have expiration dates in order to complete the study on time—for example a coupon should indicate that a recruit can be included in the study in the next two weeks. Some flexibility and judgment may be applied depending on study progress.

Bottom front of the coupon

This is the payment coupon (shown in Figure 3.2 in grey) which is used by the recruiter to claim a secondary incentive for recruiting someone. The information that it includes is:

- the name of the project
- the level of incentive for recruiting peers into the study (secondary incentive)
- the recruit's identification number

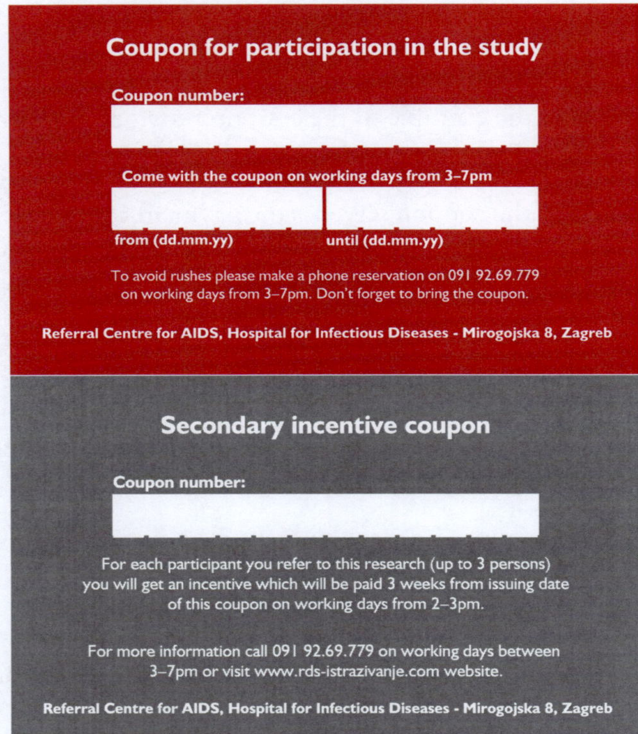

This example of a coupon is based on a RDS study among men who have sex with men carried out in Zagreb, Croatia, in 2006.

Figure 3.2 Example of the front part of the coupon

- the location of the site where the secondary incentive can be obtained, hours and telephone number (this is often the same site that a participant visited to complete a questionnaire and gave specimens).

When coming to collect the secondary incentive, a recruiter has to present the payment coupon(s).

Upper back of the coupon

The following information should be included for the recruit on the upper back part of the coupon (shown in Figure 3.3 in red):

- what tests are offered in the study and whether pre-test and post-test counselling are available
- the amount of the primary incentive given
- circumstances under which the coupon will not be accepted.

Optional:

- a map showing the location of the RDS project site so that participants can find it more easily.

Bottom back of the coupon

The bottom back part (shown in Figure 3.3 in grey) describes how a secondary incentive is administered and under what conditions secondary incentives can and cannot be given.

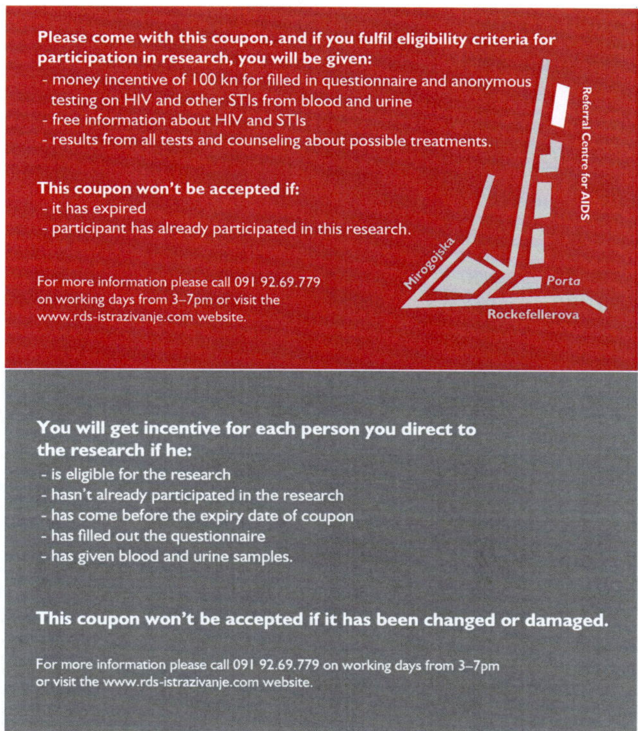

This example of a coupon is based on a RDS study among men who have sex with men carried out in Zagreb, Croatia, in 2006.

Figure 3.3 Example of the back part of the coupon

Sequential coupon numbering

The coupon system should have a numbering system that meets the needs of linking recruiter and recruit and also is easy for staff to use. Typically a sequential number can be assigned to each coupon given out by study staff. For example the third seed interviewed may get coupons 2012, 2013 and 2014. The coupons would also have the seed's unique identification number (3) on it as well. The sequential coupon number then becomes the recruit's study identification number (that is the person bringing in coupon 2012 becomes study identification number 2012). This information must be recorded in the study database as well in any coupon management database.

When claiming the secondary incentive, the following situations may occur.

- If the recruit has not enrolled in the survey, inform the recruiter and suggest that he can remind the person to whom he gave the coupon to come into the study or return to the survey site in another week to see if the person to whom he gave the coupon has enrolled in the meantime.
- If the recruit has enrolled in the survey, match the coupons in the coupon management database and give the recruiter his secondary incentive.

Situations in which the recruiter may not receive the secondary incentive

- If the expiration date on the recruitment coupons issued has passed and none of the coupons has yet been redeemed.

- If the recruiter did not bring a payment coupon.
- If the coupon appears to be fake.

The rate of coupon distribution is difficult to predict. It often happens that not all three coupons are given to target group members either because recruiters are not efficiently distributing them or potential recruits are not willing to accept coupons and participate in a survey. It is only necessary for one recruit to enrol in each wave of the study to continue the progression of a chain. In practice, some chains do not grow from initial seeds; in other cases a large part of the sample may originate from one chain. As long as equilibrium is achieved, the principle of RDS is maintained.

The sample size can be limited by tracking the recruitment chains of all seeds and stopping distribution of coupons when it has been estimated that the sample size will be soon reached. For example, when a recruitment chain reaches the third wave, interviewers can start giving two recruitment coupons instead of three. By the fifth wave, interviewers need give only one recruitment coupon, and at wave six, interviewers can stop giving coupons. The site, however, needs to remain open beyond the official end of the study, as some group members might still come to participate, and those who participated will come to collect test results and the secondary incentive. However, if recruitment goes slowly, the number of coupons distributed should not be decreased and some chains may progress to very high numbers of waves.

Step 11. Select staff

As in other surveys, there are several different responsibilities which need to be assigned to the study staff. The exact responsibilities of each staff member will depend on the local organization of the survey. It is desirable to have members of the priority population as part of the team. Some staff may take on more than one responsibility; for example, a site coordinator can take on the supervisory role.

Screeners

The screener is usually the first person with whom a potential participant will come into contact. Their tasks include:

- checking coupon validity by assessing whether the coupon is original and whether the expiration date has passed. If the coupon is not valid, the person who brought it cannot be included
- determining eligibility by asking screening questions to find out whether participants meet the inclusion criteria including not having participated in the current round of RDS. If the potential participant is not eligible or refuses to participate, the screener completes the non-eligibility form or the refusal form
- explaining the study
- performing informed consent
- stapling the coupon to the signed informed consent sheet
- explaining to participants the checklist form that they need to carry until the end of the whole process in order to get a primary incentive. The screener fills in the participant's coupon number, the study identification number and the date and checks off the box that the participant has completed the eligibility verification and has given consent for participation

- making appointments with potential respondents if they want to arrange an appointment over the phone, or if there are too many people waiting to start the screening. The screener maintains a daily appointment form, which provides dates and hours during which potential participants can come to the study site.

Interviewers (can be also VCT staff)

Interviewers

- hand out a questionnaire, set up hand-held or other computer devices, or administer a questionnaire in a face-to-face interview depending on the mode of interviewing
- record a participant's unique coupon identification number on the questionnaire
- record a participant's outgoing coupon identification numbers on the questionnaire (these are the coupons he/she will in turn give to persons in his/her social network).
- ensures the questionnaire on the network size is included in the face-to-face interview
- conduct pre- and post-test counselling (if applicable)
- tell participants when they can come to pick up the results (if applicable)
- after signing the appropriate section of the checklist form, the interviewer returns it to the participant and escorts him or her to the laboratory to give specimens (blood, urine, etc.).

Coupon manager

The coupon manager

- records coupon numbers in the coupon management database on a daily basis
- gives the coupons to a participant after writing in the correct coupon identification and the expiration date to each coupon
- manages the slowdown of the RDS coupon distribution as the survey reaches the sample size
- cooperates with the second interviewing site (if there is one) on coupon management issues
- administers primary and secondary incentives
- before giving the primary incentive, assesses the participant's checklist form to ensure that all necessary steps in data collection are completed. If the participant has missed one of the steps, then the coupon manager escorts the participant back to do the part that was missed. If the participant has completed all the steps, the coupon manager will give the primary incentive and coupons for distribution to peers
- records when the primary and secondary incentives have been paid in the financial log
- ensures that there is an adequate supply of money for incentives.

When a participant comes to collect the secondary incentive, the coupon manger completes the coupon rejecters form if the recruiter says that one or more of potential recruits would not accept a coupon. The recruiter must present the payment coupon to receive the secondary incentive. To issue the secondary incentive, the coupon manager has to check in the coupon management file whether his recruit has successfully participated in the survey.

Once the recruiter completes the coupon rejecters questionnaire, the coupon manager pays out the secondary compensation.

To avoid overcrowding, secondary incentives can be paid before the study site opens for data collection or after it finishes.

Laboratory staff and microbiologists

Laboratory staff and microbiologists

- take biological specimens (blood, urine, oral fluid) from participants
- decide on the equipment needed for testing and types of tests and arrange their purchase
- ensure biosafety of the testing room and appropriate disposal of waste
- ensure appropriate labelling, transportation and storage of samples
- ensure proper storage and quality control of test kits.

Survey coordinator

The survey coordinator

- takes the lead in planning and budgeting the study
- provides guidance on questionnaire design and organizes questionnaire piloting
- provides advice on biological specimen collection and testing
- ensures all ethical, legal and safety requirements are met
- organizes and lectures at the training course for the field staff
- ensures that there are appropriate referral pathways for HIV-positives and those who test positive for other STI
- ensures that there are procedures in place for use of universal precautions to prevent accidental transmission of pathogens
- maintains regular communication with the site manager and site staff (meetings once per week, more often if necessary)
- can participate in data analysis, interpretation of results and report writing.

Site manager

The site manager

- prepares the RDS site for data collection
- carries out day-to-day management of the site during the data collection period and makes sure that there are enough coupons, tests, questionnaires, study forms and money for incentives
- oversees the storage of biological specimens
- directs participants during the survey and ensures that all steps of data collection are completed
- liaises with the survey coordinator regarding general survey preparation issues
- identifies interviewing staff
- contributes to questionnaire piloting.

Supervisor

The supervisor

- needs to have a thorough understanding of the theory and implementation of all components of RDS, including organization of the survey, interviewing processes, coupon management and payment of incentives, and the steps involved in the collection and management of biological specimens
- sets up a meeting schedule to discuss progress and any problems during the survey. It is advisable for the supervisor to meet weekly with all the staff to address any problems and to maintain quality assurance
- oversees the performance of the interviewers, screeners and coupon manager and is responsible for ensuring that the survey protocol is strictly followed
- can fulfil the tasks of other staff member(s) if the site becomes too crowded or when a staff member is unavailable
- ensures that all documentation and questionnaires are properly filed and stored in a locked file cabinet.

If genital examinations for STI are carried out as part of the survey data collection activities, trained medical personnel must be included in the study team.

Step 12. Train site staff on RDS methods and explain staff responsibilities

All staff need to be trained on the basic principles and procedures of RDS; the organization of the site; staff responsibilities; responsibilities in administering RDS forms; handing out coupons; collecting and distributing primary and secondary incentives; working with the coupon management database; and analysis of data using the respondent-driven sampling analysis tool (RDSAT; training will only cover general aspects of RDS data analysis as the task is quite specialized).

Step 13. Decide on the levels of primary and secondary incentives

Cash is the typical type of incentive used in RDS studies, but other forms of incentive may be used, such as food vouchers, telephone cards or bus tokens. They should be determined in the formative phase and set low enough to be non-coercive but high enough to cover the costs of participation and provide some measure of incentive for participation. Once participants have completed a questionnaire and provided a biological specimen, they can receive a primary incentive. After successful recruitment of peers, they can receive the secondary incentives.

Step 14. Design the database for entering data from the questionnaire

The database for storing data from the behavioural questionnaire can be designed in any number of available software applications (e.g. Microsoft Access, SPSS, Microsoft Excel, Epi Info) and then transferred to RDSAT for analysis. A respondent-driven sampling coupon manager (RDSCM) can be downloaded, as well as RDSAT, free of charge from www.respondentdrivensampling.org and serves to record the coupon numbers. However, coupon management can be also done in a spreadsheet file and then transferred to RDSAT.

Step 15. Transfer data into RDSAT and do data analysis

That is explained briefly in chapter 5.3 on surveillance data analysis.

Step 16. Write up the report and data dissemination

Further information

Multivariate statistical analysis is not yet possible using RDSAT, and the approaches for multivariate analysis of RDS data are under development. One approach that has been used is to conduct multivariate analyses using standard statistical software and weights exported from RDSAT.

Further and more detailed information about RDS as a sampling tool and the results of the studies that used RDS are available at:

Johnston LG. *Conducting respondent-driven sampling (RDS) studies in diverse settings: a training manual for planning RDS studies*. Atlanta, Georgia, Centers for Disease Control and Prevention, 2007.

Journal of urban health, 2006, 83(1 suppl.).

RDS tools and RDSAT software are available at http://www.respondentdrivensampling.org.

3.3

Sampling for HIV surveillance in facilities

Community-based HIV surveillance surveys face many challenges in reaching the target population and logistical complexities in collecting blood and data, and have inherently high costs in time and resources. There is strong appeal, therefore, to track HIV prevalence among persons at facilities where populations at risk are seen on a routine basis and blood is already drawn for other purposes. HIV prevalence may be measured for surveillance purposes by conducting HIV testing on a sample of the patients or clients of the facilities.

For example, persons attending STI clinics are manifestly at higher risk for HIV by virtue of having an STI, having a partner with an STI and typically having multiple partners. Moreover, in many STI clinics there are high proportions of patients who are FSW, clients of FSW and MSM. TB clinics are also likely to have a high proportion of persons with HIV infection. Prisons and other detention centres have large numbers of IDU and FSW and are settings where male–male sexual behaviour may occur. STI clinics and prisons are facilities where HIV is likely to appear and be detected early in an area and are therefore considered **sentinels** for trends in the epidemic. Under the rationale that populations at risk frequent certain facilities with some stability over time, conducting annual or biennial seroprevalence surveys at such facilities (also called HIV **sentinel surveillance**) can track trends in the epidemic over time. Samples of patients or clients of these facilities are held to be "proxies" or approximations of high-risk populations from the wider community or are "sentinels" in which HIV appears early in an epidemic.

Pregnant women seen at antenatal clinics (ANC) are held to be proxies for the sexually active, general adult female population of reproductive age. Tracking HIV prevalence among women attending ANC has been a core surveillance activity in many parts of the world since the first decade of the epidemic. In generalized epidemics, HIV prevalence at ANC clinics forms the basis for making national HIV projections. Such projections, however, require broad inclusion of ANC sites nationally, including urban and rural settings, as well as periodic validation and calibration with true population-based surveys (such as the demographic and health surveys with serological HIV testing and AIDS indicator surveys). Moreover, HIV prevalence in the general population must be high enough to be able to measure with precision at ANC. Such a situation exists in parts of Sudan, Djibouti and Somalia. In low-level and concentrated HIV epidemics, such as prevail in most of the Middle East and North Africa, HIV sentinel surveillance at ANC has a more limited role. In general, ANC sentinel surveillance is recommended for large urban areas and other locations where HIV prevalence has surpassed 5% in one or more most-at-risk populations. In these settings, ANC sites serve as sentinels for bridging from most-at-risk populations to the general population.

Different facilities may serve as sentinel sites in different settings. For example, HIV prevalence among military recruits or conscripts may track the epidemic in young men as proxies of the general population (particularly if conscription is universal) or may be considered sentinel populations if many soldiers are clients of FSW. Other occupations and places of employment may also serve as sentinel populations, such as lorry and transportation companies or men employed as seamen or fishermen. In some settings, HIV testing may be universal or nearly complete and therefore provides measures of HIV prevalence without requiring conducting a special survey in a sample of the population. For example, HIV testing may be performed at some ANC sites, among military recruits upon induction or for prisoners upon intake.

Blood donors hold a cautious position as a sentinel population for HIV surveillance. On the one hand, many blood banks are (or in principle should be) conducting HIV testing on all blood donations. Therefore HIV prevalence among blood donors represents the prevalence among all potential donors, and such data should be routinely examined. However, because persons at low risk are encouraged to donate, and those at high risk or known to be infected are discouraged, such data should not be held to be a proxy of HIV prevalence for the general population. Moreover, changes in HIV prevalence among blood donors over time may reflect changes in blood banking practices, not changes in the epidemic in the area. Nonetheless, blood banks and other comprehensive testing programmes are often the largest source of HIV infection data and can be a useful signal of changes in the epidemic which may require further investigation.

In general, all HIV prevalence data from clinics and facilities require careful interpretation and continual assessment for their representativeness of the general population, their inclusion of populations at risk and changes in the make-up of the facility population over time.

How to conduct facility-based HIV surveillance is described in greater detail in other guidelines. For ANC sentinel surveillance, with discussion on TB clinics, hospitals, military, blood donors and other occupational groups, please refer to *Guidelines for conducting HIV sentinel serosurveys among pregnant women and other groups*, Geneva, UNAIDS/WHO, 2003. UNAIDS/03.49l, available at http://data.unaids.org/Publications/IRC-pub06/JC954-anc-Serosurveys_Guidelines_en.pdf. Additional guidance on HIV surveillance among TB patients can be found in *Guidelines for HIV surveillance among tuberculosis patients*. Geneva, UNAIDS/WHO, 2004. UNAIDS/04.30E, available at http://data.unaids.org/Publications/ IRC-pub06/ JC740-hiv-tb_surveillance_en.pdf.

The following section provides a brief overview and examples of approaches to HIV surveillance at facilities.

3.3.1 HIV sentinel surveillance in clinical settings (ANC, TB and STI clinics)

In clinic-based HIV surveillance, the focus is on HIV seroprevalence using leftover blood drawn for other purposes with less information on risk behaviour for several reasons.

In order to minimize bias due to patients refusing participation in HIV testing and risk behaviour surveys, HIV testing is often done at facilities as unlinked anonymous testing (UAT; see section 3.3.3 for UAT procedures). UAT permanently removes any connection of the HIV test result to the patient prior to testing. This procedure minimizes the risk to the patient through inadvertent disclosure of the test result and also does not rely on active participation of the patients. At the same time, UAT precludes the collection of detailed behavioural information for surveillance purposes, may miss opportunities to provide counselling and results to patients, and may not be deemed to meet the particular ethical standards in some countries (consult your local institutional review board or ethics committee). In some settings, informed consent is obtained to conduct UAT—HIV testing is done with patients' knowledge and permission but not linked to them individually.

Another reason why facility-based HIV sentinel surveillance collects limited behavioural data is to minimize impact on patients and clinic staff. Patients present to the clinic for reasons other than HIV surveillance (e.g. STI screening and treatment, antenatal care), and lengthy surveys may not be acceptable. Moreover, busy clinic staff do not have time to conduct detailed and good quality behavioural interviews. Facility-based HIV surveillance is therefore usually limited to abstracting the data that are already collected for other purposes. For the most part, this includes only dates, locations, basic demographic information and primary reasons for the visit.

The selection of sites to conduct HIV sentinel surveillance depends on several factors. First, geographic coverage of the facility in relation to the HIV epidemic, national priorities and representation of regions of the country may direct site selection. Second, there must be willingness and capacity on the part of clinic staff to conduct the surveillance activities entailed. Potential sites therefore need to be assessed (i.e. at pre-surveillance) on a range of issues related to successful implementation, such as staff capacities, laboratory capacities, available data, patient volume and patient flow. For each selected site, local staff and laboratory technicians need to be assigned responsibility for data abstraction and blood collection which are typically beyond their usual duties.

Another criterion for including sites is whether they can achieve the sample size required—whether patient volume is sufficient in a short period of time. The sample size can be calculated per site or per certain area by aggregating specific sites (e.g. for more remote areas, inclusion of satellite clinics). Sample size calculations are explained in more detail below. For surveillance, HIV prevalence is usually tracked over time across each site and/or region and by the median for the country as a whole.

3.3.2   Steps in data collection in clinic-based surveillance

Clinic-based surveillance can be divided into two phases:

- phase 1 preparation: pre-surveillance assessment, selection of clinics and preparation of survey instruments and sites
- phase 2 implementation: surveillance data collection.

Phase 1. Pre-surveillance assessment, selection of clinics and preparation of survey instruments and sites

Pre-surveillance assessment comprises three steps.

Step 1 includes defining eligibility criteria for inclusion of clinics, establishment of a list of all eligible clinics, the selection of clinics for pre-surveillance assessment and verification of selected clinics for suitability.

Suggested eligibility criteria for inclusion of clinics include:

- geographic location (urban, peri-urban, rural)—typically one or two sites (one urban and one rural) are selected per province or district. Ideally, clinics to be included in a national HIV surveillance system would be randomly selected in order to approximate representativeness of the country. However, in practice, this is rarely feasible as the number of suitable sites may be severely limited in some regions. Moreover, a rationale for most sentinel surveillance systems is to create a network of sites that is able to detect the appearance of HIV infection and trends in HIV prevalence in different parts of the country. Therefore, criteria such as a minimum geographic coverage of all areas of the country, number of clients and willingness and capabilities of staff predominate in the selection of sites
- number of clients/patients seen per day (and per month) so that estimates can be made about the duration of data collection and the potential sample size per site. The site should provide services to a sufficiently large number of attendees who meet eligibility criteria in order to reach the required sample size within a reasonable timeframe (for example 30 clients/patients per week would achieve a sample of 300 in 10 weeks)
- number of staff (nurses, doctors, laboratory technicians)
- number and type of patients from whom blood samples are routinely taken.

Based on these criteria a list of eligible clinics is produced that can be stratified by region and urban and rural location (Table 3.5). From this list, a final set of clinics is selected for pre-surveillance to be visited and assessed for their suitability and readiness to be included in the HIV surveillance activities. In addition to the above, criteria for final inclusion include:

- types of on-site services available (family planning, voluntary HIV counselling and testing, prevention of mother-to-child transmission); of note, the availability of on-site voluntary HIV testing is often considered an ethical criterion for including the site in HIV surveillance, particularly when UAT is being done
- geographic balance (urban, peri-urban, rural), typically one or two sites (one urban and one rural) should be selected per province or district
- ability to describe the catchment area the clinic serves (e.g. rural, peri-urban, urban or particular area)

Table 3.5 Characteristics of the sites selected for clinic-based HIV surveillance

No.	Name of site	Region	Urban/peri-urban/rural	Demonstrated high-risk area for HIV*	Provider (public or private)	Facility (hospital or OPD†)	Patient load per week	Easily reachable for supervision
1								
2								
3								
4								
5								
6								
7								
8								
9								
10								
11								
12								

*   Categories can include: low, medium, high, unknown.

†   OPD = outpatient department.

- ability to describe the populations that the clinic serves (e.g. any high inclusion of most-at-risk populations)
- number and type of patients from whom blood samples are routinely taken
- possibility of storing specimens, and duration of storage; availability of electricity and whether shortages occur; if so, how often and whether a generator is available
- whether blood can be regularly sent to the laboratory where HIV testing is performed, and whether there are any problems that could happen with specimen collection and transport
- whether the clinic has any other factors that may influence the client population, e.g. is there a fee that patients need to pay to visit that health care site? Has this changed over time?

In countries with generalized epidemics where a considerable proportion of the population lives in rural areas, rural ANC clinics need to be selected for surveillance to obtain national-level estimates of HIV prevalence. Selection criteria for rural sites can include:

- located more than 50 km from an urban centre or major road
- located in a village with a population not exceeding a certain number of inhabitants (number to be defined by each country)
- more than 75% of the site's catchment population generate their income through agriculture.

Laboratories where testing will be done should be selected according to the following criteria:

- willingness to participate
- technical capacity to conduct the study
- qualification of technical staff
- routine performance of relevant tests
- quality assurance programmes in place
- waste disposal facility.

In low-level and concentrated HIV epidemics, selection of clinics should prioritize high-risk areas and client populations with high numbers of most-at-risk populations to serve as an early warning system to detect increases in HIV prevalence and potential bridging to other populations.

The information on potential clinical surveillance sites should be recorded in a form such as Table 3.5 for monitoring the process of data collection and for data interpretation.

Step 2 comprises development, field-testing and finalization of surveillance data collection forms. With UAT, only data that are already collected and recorded in patient records are to be abstracted. A short data abstraction form that contains the necessary and available demographic (and in some cases limited behavioural) data should be developed and pilot-tested.

Step 3 comprises training of clinic and surveillance staff on the surveillance protocol, including the provision of operational procedures for data collection in writing. The topics to be covered during training on clinic-based HIV surveillance are listed below.

Principles of surveillance	Definition of surveillance
	HIV surveillance
	Objectives of sentinel surveillance survey
	How data will be used for planning HIV and STI prevention and control programmes
Survey design	Selection of clinics
	Selection of patients
	Principles of unlinked anonymous testing
	Ethics of data collection
	Importance of adhering to protocols
Data collection	Data collection forms
	Unlinking blood specimens and data collection forms
	Testing for HIV and storage of blood specimens
	Sending data to surveillance focal points
Blood tests	HIV tests and tests for syphilis
	Other blood tests that will be performed
Supervision	Eligibility criteria
	Sampling process
	Completeness of data collection forms
	Labelling of blood specimens
	Storage of blood specimens
	Transfer of data to the surveillance office for analysis

Phase 2. Implementation phase: surveillance data collection

In phase 2, surveillance data are collected by selecting patients using either **consecutive sampling**, **systematic sampling** or **random sampling**.

Consecutive sampling consists of selecting every patient who meets the inclusion criteria during the time of data collection until the desired sample size is reached. Systematic sampling consists of making a list of every patient who meets the inclusion criteria, and then selecting every nth (for example, every third or fourth) from the list until the required sample size is reached. Systematic sampling also starts with a randomly selected number, then counting out the interval for inclusion. Simple random sampling uses a random number table or other method (for instance, a computer-based method) to generate a list of random numbers. These numbers are then matched with a list of patients who meet the eligibility criteria.

Systematic and random sampling are more likely to produce representative samples. However, consecutive sampling is the preferred method for clinic-based HIV surveillance sampling as it is easy to employ and reduces the likelihood of error and bias created by clinic staff in selecting patients.

It is recommended that data be collected during a period of eight to 12 weeks, though this might be extended to up to six months, depending on the number of patients attending and the required sample size.

If HIV testing is done as UAT, the blood used for HIV testing is taken from the remnant blood that was collected for other routine diagnostic procedures. Most commonly, the blood used for HIV testing was originally drawn for syphilis testing, particularly for STI patients and pregnant women, which is offered to *all* patients attending the site as part of routine care, regardless of eligibility for the survey.

The methods of UAT require complete separation of information for surveillance from the routine care ongoing at the selected sites. To accomplish this, two patient identification numbers are used: one for the named, linked diagnostic tests and the other for the unlinked anonymous test. The UAT code can have a format that is agreed upon in the country—for example it can consist of the number format *xx-yyy-zzzz: xx* in this case defines the sentinel site, and remains unchanged for all specimens originating from the corresponding site. *yyy* is a number that is unique for every woman or man sampled at that site and *zzzz* denotes the year. It can be pre-printed on self-adhesive labels or written down. Numbers that are used for coding patients can be generated randomly by programs such as MS Excel or Stata or from the web (see: http://www.random.org/).

Other data that are abstracted from clinic records usually include age and/or date of birth, gravidity (at ANC clinics), marital status, residence (urban/rural), educational level and occupation. A data abstraction form for HIV surveillance survey using UAT is available in appendix 3.10. Note that according to ethical guidelines for UAT, only data that are already routinely collected from patients may be abstracted.

The key step in UAT is that HIV testing is only conducted after all identifying information and any means of linking the UAT number to a clinic identification number have been permanently destroyed. This ensures that HIV test results can never be associated with individuals. Steps on how this is accomplished are provided below, and more detail is provided in *Guidelines for conducting HIV sentinel serosurveys among pregnant women and other groups*. Geneva, UNAIDS/WHO, 2003. UNAIDS/03.49l, available at http://data.unaids.org/Publications/IRC-pub06/JC954-anc-Serosurveys_Guidelines_en.pdf.

3.3.3 Procedures for unlinked anonymous HIV testing (UAT)

The key advantage of UAT is that there is no bias resulting from clinic patients refusing to have an HIV test result, therefore producing true estimates of HIV prevalence in the clinic population. HIV test results in UAT are permanently delinked from individuals and therefore not revealed to patients and are not available to the staff. For ethical reasons, patients at the selected surveillance sites should have the opportunity to be tested for HIV through the site's own voluntary testing programme or at other sites nearby if they want to know their HIV status.

The UAT methods requires that all personal identification be removed prior to HIV testing and that any new patient identifiers made for the purposes of surveillance cannot be linked to indentifying information or clinic patient id numbers.

The UAT methods also require that no new blood be drawn for the purposes of surveillance, but rather that leftover blood from other routine tests be used. Once the laboratory receives the specimen, laboratory personnel will spin down the serum. HIV testing is done by transferring an aliquot of 0.5–2.0 ml of leftover serum from syphilis or other testing to a sterile plastic tube or a cryovial. Ideally, aliquoted specimens should be stored at –20 °C [6]. Serum can be stored at 2–5 °C at the site for up to three days. For longer-term storage (e.g. years), specimens should be stored at –70 °C. For longer storage periods, sera should be aliquoted before storage because repeatedly freezing and thawing the same sample to draw off aliquots degrades the sample and may produce erroneous results. If there is no refrigerator in the health facility or if for any other reason the storage of the samples cannot be done at the facility, specimens need to be transported to another place using a cold box and ice bags.

UAT for HIV surveillance is typically done at a central laboratory away from the clinic itself. This is usually a regional or national reference laboratory. This ensures standardization and quality assurance for test results. It also provides another delinking from the clinic staff.

On-site HIV UAT

To ensure patient anonymity, the following steps need to be performed by different staff when testing is done on site.

1. Staff member 1 collects the blood from a patient and labels it with a standard clinic code.
2. Staff member 1 labels a standard clinic form with the same code and records on that form the routinely collected demographic and clinical information about a patient.
3. Staff member 1 removes one aliquot of blood and puts it in a second tube and labels it with a new code (that is, a UAT code). The blood specimen in this tube is used for UAT.
4. Staff member 1 records the necessary demographic and clinical data on the surveillance form for UAT. Staff member 1 records also the new code used for UAT on that form. This surveillance form does not have any personal information that can identify a patient. Staff member 1 sends the surveillance form for UAT to the regional/national surveillance institution.
5. Staff member 1 sends the tube with the UAT code to staff member 2, who performs the HIV test. At this point, there is no linkage of the UAT code number to the standard clinic code number.
6. The UAT code is not recorded in any place where it could be traced back to the patient or to the clinic code number.
7. Staff member 2 sends the results of HIV UAT with codes to the regional/national surveillance institution.
8. The demographic and clinical data from the surveillance forms and the results of HIV UAT are linked by UAT codes and analysed at the regional/national surveillance institution. The regional/national surveillance institution is in charge of data collection from all participating sentinel sites.

In on-site testing, in order to ensure patient anonymity it is important that:

- one staff member performs the routine clinical testing
- another staff member performs UAT for HIV.

In on-site testing, a separate laboratory log book is used to record results from UAT.

Off-site HIV UAT

An alternative approach, which ensures anonymity, particularly at small clinical sites, is to send specimens for UAT off-site to a regional or national laboratory. Clinical forms coded with UAT codes are sent to the regional/national surveillance institutions. A regional/national laboratory sends the HIV test results linked with UAT codes to the regional/national surveillance institution where they are linked with surveillance forms and analysed.

In the Middle East and North Africa, this approach is more frequently used as clinics usually do not have facilities to do HIV testing on-site. Off-site testing at a selected laboratory for all sentinel sites is also better from the point of quality assurance and standardization. The proper transport of specimens is extremely important.

3.3.4 Supervision

Supervision should be carried out at least twice per month at each site during data collection, depending on organizational and logistical issues. During supervision, the following issues need to be assessed and documented and will be also helpful for interpretation of results.

- Are survey protocols and standard operating procedures available in writing to all staff involved in data collection? Are data collection staff able to describe and explain the procedures?
- Are there any problems with inclusion of patients? How many patients who met the inclusion criteria were not included? What were the reasons for exclusion, including refusal to give blood for syphilis testing; the clinic was too busy; any other reason?
- Were there any problems with specimen collection and storage? How many times did electricity shortages occur and how did that affect storage of samples?
- Are all data collection forms properly filled in? Supervisors need to look at the forms and identify missing data.
- If HIV testing is performed using rapid HIV tests, are there sufficient test kits in storage, are they stored properly, and their dates of use valid?
- Is serum and/or whole blood stored at the appropriate temperature?
- How do laboratory staff carry out and interpret HIV rapid test results?

3.3.5 ANC clinics as sentinel sites

HIV serosurveillance among pregnant women is a core surveillance activity in countries with generalized epidemics. In generalized epidemics, trends in HIV prevalence among women attending ANC are considered as a proxy for trends in HIV prevalence in the general population, particularly when calibrated against data from population-based surveys [7, 8]. However, ANC clinics may not be truly representative of the general population, and there are several potential sources of bias. For example, accessibility of ANC clinics may be low in some countries (such as Somalia and Sudan), ANC attendance may be low when women tend to deliver at home, there may be differences in who attends and who delivers at home, or population mobility may be high and therefore attendees may not represent the population of the area.

In low-level and concentrated epidemics, ANC serosurveillance should be limited to large cities, areas where HIV prevalence has exceeded 5% in any most-at-risk population, border areas, main highways and areas where there are groups at higher risk of HIV such as most-at-risk populations or migrants from high prevalence countries.

In interpreting ANC sentinel surveillance data, high importance is placed on HIV prevalence among young women (15–24 years) as infection in this age group is more likely to be recent and therefore may be used as a proxy for HIV incidence. However, caution is needed as the sample size for this younger age group may be small.

Objectives of HIV sentinel surveillance at ANC clinics

- To estimate and compare HIV prevalence among pregnant women in the selected ANC sites and regionally and nationally (depending on the survey's design, population can be divided into strata according to residence: urban, peri-urban or rural). The median site-specific prevalence should be reported, together with median for regions (with range), and median for the country (with range). If a mean prevalence is calculated, then estimates need to account for the underlying differences in population sizes served by the sites; that is, standardized rates should be calculated if the aim is to obtain regional estimates. The EPP package (see below) is one means of calculating such standardized rates.
- To monitor trends in HIV prevalence over time.
- To estimate HIV prevalence according to age group: 15–24; 25–34; 35–49 (if the sample size permits, 15–19 and 20–24 should be analysed separately).
- To assess the sociodemographic profile of sentinel site attendees in order to facilitate interpretation of HIV prevalence estimates.

Inclusion criteria for HIV sentinel surveillance at ANC clinics

- Pregnant women attending the clinic for the first time during their current pregnancy during the serosurvey period.
- Aged 15–49 years.
- Acceptance of syphilis testing if HIV testing is carried out as UAT.

The key outcomes of data analysis

- HIV prevalence per site (and per region or district).
- Trends in HIV prevalence over time.
- Estimation of the regional/national HIV prevalence levels (note: extrapolation of ANC site-specific data to national estimates is done through the EPP or Epidemic Projection Package software, available at http://www.unaids.org/en/knowledgecentre/HIVdata/ epidemiology/epi_software2007.asp).
- HIV prevalence stratified by the following age groups: 15–24; 25–34; 35–49. If the sample size permits, data can be stratified by age groups 15–19 and 20–24.

- HIV prevalence stratified by other sociodemographic characteristics.
- HIV prevalence by urban, peri-urban and rural strata.

Stratification is usually only feasible where HIV prevalence is high or the sample size is very large.

It is recommended that the survey be repeated every other year if HIV prevalence is more than 1%. Depending on the findings and resources available, ANC sites can be expanded to other high-risk areas of the country in subsequent years.

A data abstraction form for an HIV surveillance survey based on UAT at ANC clinics is available in appendix 3.10.

3.3.6 TB clinics as sentinel sites

TB is the most common opportunistic infection associated with HIV, and the HIV epidemic continues to fuel the TB epidemic. HIV surveillance among TB patients therefore estimates the impact of HIV on the TB epidemic, provides a marker for trends in HIV-related morbidity and is a means for planning of care and treatment in those co-infected with HIV and TB. HIV prevalence among TB patients is also an indicator of the maturity of the HIV epidemic. HIV prevalence is usually higher among those who are smear-negative or with extrapulmonary tuberculosis. If HIV testing is a routine part of TB patient management, as suggested for generalized HIV epidemics, then TB notification forms can be expanded to include HIV status, which can lead to establishment of a routine HIV surveillance system among TB patients.

Inclusion criteria for HIV sentinel surveillance at TB clinics

- Newly diagnosed TB patients attending the clinic during the serosurvey period (note: if HIV testing of all TB patients is routine, then UAT for a sampling period may not be needed).
- Patients aged 18–59 years (the age limit can be lower or higher, depending on the survey design and characteristics of the epidemic).
- Acceptance of other blood testing if HIV testing is carried out as UAT.

Objectives and outcomes of analysis are similar to those for ANC clinics described above. A data collection form for an HIV surveillance survey based on UAT at TB clinics is available in appendix 3.11.

3.3.7 STI clinics as sentinel sites

STI clinics are useful sentinel sites in all stages of an HIV epidemic as attendees usually have high levels of sexual risk behaviour and include many most-at-risk populations (FSW, clients of FSW, MSM, persons with multiple sex partners). After ANC clinics, STI clinics may be the most common sites for clinic-based HIV surveillance.

However, there are many challenges in conducting STI clinic HIV sentinel surveillance in the Middle East and North Africa. In many parts of the region, STI clinics either do not exist as separate clinics, are poorly attended or serve other care purposes as well. For example, gynaecological outpatient departments can serve as STI sites, in which case data must record the purpose of the visit. Patients may be women coming for family planning and contraception advice or suffering from a range of gynaecological disorders and are therefore not STI patients. Along a similar line, dermato-venerological clinics might be attended mainly by dermatological patients, without adequate numbers of patients with STI symptoms. A suggestion for these situations is to conduct HIV surveillance with only male patients with urethral discharge and male and female patients with genital ulcer disease, as they are highly likely to be caused by sexually transmitted pathogens. Another challenge in the region is that many people with STI-related symptoms self-treat or attend private clinics. All these factors contribute to the challenge of having a sufficient number of true STI patients at these sites to meet the sample size needed for HIV sentinel surveillance and in the interpretation of data.

Inclusion criteria for HIV sentinel surveillance in STI patients[1]

- Men with urethral discharge.
- Men and women with genital ulcers.

or

- All those diagnosed with STI. This may include patients with syndromic and/ or etiological STI diagnosis with or without symptoms, depending on the STI case definition used for the purpose of the survey.

and

- Acceptance of routine blood testing if HIV testing is carried out as UAT.

It would be useful to have "reason for attendance" and "presence of symptoms" as variables on the data collection form for this type of surveillance, because this will give a clearer picture about the types of patient that attend the clinic.

Objectives and outcomes of analysis are similar to ANC clinics described above. A data collection form for an HIV surveillance survey based on UAT at STI clinics is available in appendix 3.12.

---

[1] This implies that patients are selected based on the syndromic management approach. Etiological STI testing is often not done in resource-poor countries due to lack of equipment and testing facilities.

3.4

Sample size

A sample size calculation is an essential part of planning a surveillance survey. It aims to demonstrate that the proposed study is capable of answering the objectives and questions posed. The sample size determines the precision of our estimates, which is typically expressed as a 95% confidence interval. The wider the confidence interval, the less precise the estimate. For example, if the 95% confidence interval of the point prevalence estimate of HIV of 8% is 6%–12%, it means that there is 95% probability that the true population prevalence lies between 6% and 12%. If we repeated the study 100 times, in 95 cases we would expect the prevalence estimates to be between 6% and 12%. As a rule, more precision or narrower confidence intervals will require larger sample sizes.

The calculation of the sample size for HIV surveillance surveys is usually based on the desired precision around our estimate of HIV prevalence or around key behavioural measures. Because surveillance is an ongoing activity that tracks trends over time, sample size calculations are also made accounting for changes in prevalence over time or from one year's survey to the next.

This section provides a template for calculating a simple sample size in community-based surveys. Consultation with a statistician is recommended for more complex surveys and for designing national surveillance systems.

The key ingredients for a sample size estimate in a community-based survey are:

- estimated prevalence of the key outcome(s) in a target population (behavioural or biological)
- estimated change in the prevalence of this key outcome over time (in order to be able to assess trends)
- level of significance (p value)
- level of power
- the statistical test used.

For the level of significance (p value), it is common practice to use $p < 0.05$ as indicating that there is substantial evidence that the null hypothesis is untrue[1]. A p value of less than 0.05 is often reported as "statistically significant", which reflects an arbitrary decision

---

[1] Research studies are based on testing hypotheses and require a statement of the hypothesis that will be tested, which is usually called the null hypothesis. It represents the assertion that there is no relationship between exposure and outcome. The p value should be considered as a guide to the likelihood that chance is an explanation of the findings. From Hennekens CH, Buring JE. *Epidemiology in medicine.* Philadelphia, Lippincott, Williams & Williams, 1987.

that a 5% probability is small enough to suggest that the observed result is due to chance. The *p* value is derived to test the null hypothesis that there is no association between exposure and the outcome variable [25]. For example, a *p* value of 0.02 means that there is a probability of 0.02 (2% chance) that a result of the observed magnitude or greater could have occurred by chance alone and not because of a real difference.

The power of the study is the probability that we will find a predetermined magnitude of change in the measure, if the change really happened. It is conventionally set at 80%, which means that we can be 80% certain that our sample was large enough to detect a change of the predetermined magnitude or greater.

The formula used for sample size calculation depends on the statistical test used for analysis. In cross-sectional HIV surveillance studies, we often base calculations of the sample size on comparison of two proportions, and this approach will be presented in these guidelines. However, sample size calculations can be also done based on the precision around a single proportion, mean or rate; an odds ratio; or comparisons of two means, two proportions or two rates.

3.4.1   Formula for calculating the sample size for a cross-sectional survey with one round of data[1]

The formula for calculating the sample size *n* for only one survey round is based on the width of the confidence interval desired; that is, the precision or the margin of error considered acceptable (for example, ±3%, which is the same as a total width of 6%) [26]. The desired precision of the estimate specifies that the estimated prevalence should not differ from the real prevalence by more than *d* percentage points with 95% confidence.

$$n = \frac{Z_{1-\alpha}^{2}\, P(1-P)}{d^{2}} \times D$$

where n = sample size

$Z_{1-\alpha}$ is a factor that corresponds to the desired significance level (for a 5% significance level, $Z_{1-\alpha}$ = 1.96)

P is the estimated prevalence (for example, prevalence of HIV)

d is the required precision (or the margin of error considered acceptable)

D = design effect.

Example 1. In addition to the margin of error, cluster-based surveys need to account for the design effect in their sample size estimations. The design effect is based on how similar people are within the cluster compared to overall. As an example, we are conducting a cluster-based survey and we want the estimated HIV prevalence (in this example taken as 5%) to be within 2 percentage points of the true population prevalence with 95% confidence. The value of design effect for cluster-based survey is taken as 2.

$$n = \frac{1.96^{2} \times 0.05 \times (1-0.05)}{0.02^{2}} \times 2 = 456 \times 2 = 912$$

---

[1]   Source: *Guidelines for measuring national HIV prevalence in population-based surveys.* Geneva, UNAIDS/WHO Working Group on Global HIV/AIDS and STI surveillance, 2005.

Table 3.5 Sample size for a given HIV prevalence and level of precision

Precision[*]	Prevalence								
	1%	2%	3%	4%	5%	10%	15%	20%	25%
±0.5%	3 042	6 024	8 943	11 801	14 598	27 660	39 184	49 172	57 624
±1%	760	1 506	2 236	2 950	3 649	6 914	9 796	12 293	14 406
±2%		376	559	738	912	1 729	2 449	3 073	3 601
±3%			248	328	405	768	1 088	1 366	1 601
±4%				184	228	432	612	768	900
±5%					146	277	392	492	576
±10%							69	98	123	144

* Precision is related to the width of the confidence interval. For example, the minimum sample size for ANC-based sentinel surveillance calculated by taking into account the prevalence of HIV of 2% and 2% precision is 376. If precision is set higher, for example at 1%, then the desired sample size is 1506 respondents.

Table 3.5 shows the approximate sample sizes based on the above formula, taking into account the baseline prevalence, desired precision and a design effect of 2. The adjustment for the non-response should be done separately.

3.4.2 Formula for calculating the sample size to detect a change in the prevalence over two survey rounds[1]

This is the formula for the sample size calculations when the purpose is to assess change in the indicator over two rounds of surveillance surveys.

$$n = \frac{\left[Z_{1-\alpha}\sqrt{2P(1-P)} + Z_{1-\beta}\sqrt{P_1(1-P_1) + P_2(1-P_2)} \right]^2}{\Delta^2} \times D$$

where D = design effect (see section 3.4.4 below)

P_1 = the estimated proportion at the time of the first survey round

P_2 = the estimated proportion at the future survey round

$P = (P_1 + P_2)/2$

$\Delta = P_2 - P_1$

$Z_{1-\alpha}$ = the Z-score corresponding to desired level of significance, that is percentage of the normal distribution corresponding to the required significance level. If the level of significance (α) is 5%, then the value of the one-tailed Z-score is 1.645 and of the two-tailed Z-score 1.960. The value of $Z_{1-\alpha}$ can be based on either a

---

1 Source: *Behavioral surveillance surveys. Guidelines for repeated behavioral surveys in populations at risk of HIV.* Durham, North Carolina, Family Health International, 2000.

one-tailed test or a two-tailed test. A two-tailed test is usually preferred as it enables one to detect change in both directions (either an increase or a decrease) but requires a larger sample size.

$Z_{1-\beta}$ = the Z-score corresponding to the desired level of power; that is the percentage point of the normal distribution corresponding to 100%—the power (power = 90%), $Z_{1-\beta}$ = 1.282.

The change in the indicator that we want to measure will depend on the objectives of the national response in terms of reducing HIV prevalence or risk behaviour. For surveillance, it is generally recommended that a target of 10–15 percentage points be taken as an estimate of a change in the behavioural indicators. If the baseline level of the indicator is not known, the recommended value of P_1 should be 50% (for example, 50% condom use as the baseline) as this will produce the most conservative sample size (i.e. largest that may be needed)[1].

Example 2. As an example, let us assume that we want to do a behavioural surveillance survey among IDU, and data from a baseline survey show that 55% of them shared needles at the most recent injection. Suppose that we want to be able to detect a decrease in sharing of needles of 10 percentage points. Thus, P_1 is set at 0.55 and P_2 at 0.45. We decide to choose the level of significance of 5% ($Z_{1-\alpha}$ = 1.96) and power of 90% ($Z_{1-\beta}$ = 1.282). That means that our survey has 90% power to detect a change of 10 percentage points, either a decrease or an increase. The calculation of the sample size is:

$$n = \frac{\left[\left(1.96\sqrt{2 \times 0.5 \times 0.5}\right) + 1.28\sqrt{\left(0.55 \times 0.45\right) + \left(0.45 \times 0.55\right)}\right]^2}{\left(0.45 - 0.55\right)^2} \times 2$$

$$n = 2 \times (1.386 + 0.900)^2/0.01 = 1046 \text{ injection drug users}$$

The large sample size in this case is due to the small change that we would like to be able to detect (10%).

3.4.3 Adjustment for non-response

The calculated sample size should be increased to allow for possible non-response. All surveys should strive to keep the non-response as low as possible (e.g. < 5%); however, it is wise to plan for possible higher non-response (25%, for example). If we estimate that x% of people will not respond, the sample size should be multiplied by $100/(100 - x)$. For example, if x = 25%, the multiplying factor should be $100/(100 - 25)$ = 1.33. Therefore, to incorporate an anticipated level of non-response, the sample sizes calculated by the formulas and tables noted above need to be increased accordingly.

Example 3. As an example of adjusting for non-response, example 3 adds this element to the numbers from example 1. In example 1, we calculated a required sample size of 912. To take response rate into consideration, let us assume a response rate to the questionnaire of 90% and an HIV test response rate of 80% (this gives an overall response rate of 0.9 × 0.8 = 0.72, or a non-response rate of 0.28). For the above calculation, the overall sample size after considering the response rate of 0.72 is 912/0.72 = 1267. Of note, a 28% non-response rate is substantial, and efforts should be made to maximize participation.

---

[1]   This is because variances of indicators measured as proportions are maximized at 50%.

3.4.4 Adjustment for clustered designs

In studies that employ randomized clusters rather than simple random sampling of individuals, sample size needs to be increased by a factor known as **design effect**. The Design effect depends on the **intraclass correlation coefficient** (ICC), which is the ratio of the between-cluster variance to the total variance. This is because individuals within a cluster are usually more similar to each other than to individuals in other clusters. Design effects will be larger if the number of individuals per cluster is large and if the intraclass correlation coefficient is large.

$$\text{Design effect } D = 1 + ([n' - 1] \times \text{ICC})$$

where n' = average number of individuals per cluster.

A correction for a design effect is needed in multi-stage cluster sampling design. Its value is calculated based on the variations in behaviour within and between PSU. Assuming the sizes of PSU are relatively small compared to the overall sample (e.g. 10 individuals within 30 clusters), the value of D can be generally kept at 2.0 as a rule of thumb. RDS also entails a design effect, with default values often higher than 2.0. A design effect of 2 means that the variance of cluster sampling is twice that of simple random sampling of individuals, and will double the sample size needed. Design effect = 1 in simple random sampling.

3.4.5 Other considerations in sample size calculations

In general, sample sizes usually run in the range of several hundred for most-at-risk population surveys (sex workers, MSM, IDU), to more than 1000 individuals for lower-risk groups and in household-based surveys (youth, general population). In stratified sampling, random samples have to be selected from each stratum. For information on how to calculate sample size for each stratum see: *Guidelines for measuring national HIV prevalence in population-based surveys*. Geneva, UNAIDS/WHO Working Group on Global HIV/AIDS and STI surveillance, 2005. Available at http://www.who.int/hiv/pub/surveillance/measuring/en/index.html.

The STATCALC feature of Epi Info software provides a user-friendly sample-size calculator for setting specific target sample sizes.

Readers who are interested in understanding in greater detail the statistical background of the sample size calculations are advised to read textbooks on statistics, such as:

- Kirkwood BR, Sterne JAC. *Medical statistics*, 2nd ed. Oxford, Blackwell Science, 2003.
- Stroup DF, Teutsch SM. *Statistics in public health. Quantitative approaches to public health problems*. Oxford, Oxford University Press, 1998.

Appendix 3

Forms for clusters for use in the field

Forms used in respondent-driven sampling

Data collection forms used in HIV sentinel surveillance in ANC, TB and STI clinics

Forms for clusters for use in the field

Appendix 3.1

PSU selection sheet: probability proportional to size approach

Subpopulation _______________________Geographic location ___________________

PSU NUMBER[1]	PSU NAME	MEASURE OF SIZE	CUMULATIVE SIZE	SAMPLE SELECTION NUMBER[2]	MARK THE PSU SELECTED
1					
2					
3					
4					
5					
6					
7					
8					
9					
10					
11					
12					
13					
14					
15					
Continues					

Source: *Behavioral surveillance surveys. Guidelines for repeated behavioral surveys in populations at risk of HIV.* Durham, North Carolina, Family Health International, 2000.

Do the following steps:

1. Calculate total cumulative measure of size: ____

2. Calculate sampling interval (total cumulative measure of size/number of PSU that we want to select): ____

3. Select random start number (random number between 1 and sampling interval):[3] ___________

4. Write which PSU were selected: ____

____

Note. In selecting the PSU, it is important to retain the decimal points in the sampling interval. When the decimal part of the sample selection number is less than 0.5, the lower-numbered PSU is chosen, and when it is greater than or equal to 0.5, the higher-numbered PSU is chosen.

---

[1]   Continues until the last PSU is recorded.
[2]   That is calculated by adding random start number (RS + SI, RS + 2SI, RS + 3SI, etc.).
[3]   The unit within whose cumulated measure of size this random number falls is the first unit for sampling. Subsequent units are chosen by adding the SI to this random number. This is followed until the list has been exhausted.

Appendix 3.2

PSU selection sheet: equal probability of selection approach

Subpopulation _________________________Geographic location _____________________

PSU NUMBER	PSU NAME	SAMPLE SELECTION NUMBER	MARK THE PSU SELECTED
1			
2			
3			
4			
5			
6			
7			
8			
9			
10			
11			
12			
13			
14			
15			
Continues			

Source: *Behavioral surveillance surveys. Guidelines for repeated behavioral surveys in populations at risk of HIV.* Durham, North Carolina, Family Health International, 2000.

Do the following steps:

1. Total number of PSU: ____

2. Planned number of PSU: ____

3. Calculate sampling interval (total number of PSU/planned number of PSU): _______________

4. Select random start number (random number between 1 and sampling interval)[1]: ___________

5. Write which PSU were selected: ____

____

[1] PSU that corresponds to this random number is selected as the first PSU in the sample. Subsequent units are selected by adding the SI to the random sampling number (RS + SI, RS + 2SI, RS + 3SI, etc.).

Appendix 3.3

Cluster information sheet

This form should be completed for each cluster included in sampling. The information collected will be used to calculate the sampling probabilities and sample weights before the analysis and will enable the non-response rate to be estimated.

It is important because of the following reasons:

- the estimated measure of size was obtained during mapping and sampling frame development, but on the date of the survey we might obtain a different measure of size (that is referred to as actual measure of size)
- we need to estimate how many people refused to participate
- we need to know the number of duplicates (particularly if the population is mobile)
- we need to know the number of people who completed the interviews

Geographic location ___________________________

Interviewer name ___________________________

PSU number/name ___________________________

Date and time when PSU is visited ___________________________

Estimated measure of size (before the survey) ___________________________

Actual measure of size (on the day of the survey) ___________________________

Number of people approached to be interviewed ___________________________

Number of people refused to be interviewed ___________________________

Number of duplicates ___________________________

Number of interviews completed ___________________________

Number of those ineligible ___________________________

Number of people who received incentives ___________________________

Amount of incentive given ___________________________

Forms used in respondent-driven sampling

The forms listed provide examples only and should be adapted to the target groups surveyed, eligibility criteria and design and organizational characteristics of a local RDS

Appendix 3.4

Client checklist form

Instructions. This is a form that is given to participants by a screener. A participant carries it throughout the whole process of data collection at the site, and gives it to the appropriate staff member at each step of data collection. A staff member then signs to verify that a participant completed each of the steps in data collection.

Date of interview		
Coupon number		
Survey identification number		
	Tick ✓ or ✗	**Staff signature**
Eligible to participate[1]	Yes ☐ No ☐	
Consent given[2]	Yes ☐ No ☐	
Form on the network size completed	Yes ☐ No ☐	
Behavioural questionnaire completed	Yes ☐ No ☐	
Following biological specimens given:		
• blood	Yes ☐ No ☐	
• urine	Yes ☐ No ☐	
• oral fluid	Yes ☐ No ☐	
• anal/rectal swab	Yes ☐ No ☐	
• vaginal/cervical swab	Yes ☐ No ☐	
Recruitment coupons given	Yes ☐ No ☐	
Primary incentive given	Yes ☐ No ☐	
Secondary incentive given:		
First	Yes ☐ No ☐	
Second	Yes ☐ No ☐	
Third	Yes ☐ No ☐	
Comments:		

---

[1] If a participant is not eligible, fill out non-eligibility form.
[2] If a participant does not want to give consent, fill out the refuse to participate form.

Appendix 3.5

Size of the network form (essential for the RDS analysis)

Instructions. These questions should be read to the participant by an interviewer.

1. How many other sex workers[1] do you know by name and they know you and your name, they live in the same area/city, and you have seen them in the past three months[2]?

    ____

2. How many of those women you mentioned are[3]:

    a. under the age of 18[4]? _______________________________________

3. How many women that you mentioned in Question 1 and who are older than 18 years will you consider when distributing the coupons?

    ____

4. The person who gave you a coupon is your:

    a. friend

    b. acquaintance

    c. sex partner

    d. relative

    e. I saw that person for the first time when he or she gave me the coupon

5. Why did you accept the coupon and decide to participate in this study?

    a. because of an incentive

    b. because I wanted to be tested for HIV

    c. Because I wanted to be tested for STI

    d. because I wanted to have HIV testing and counselling

    e. I was persuaded to participate by my peers

    f. the study seems to be interesting and useful

    g. because I had time to spend

    h. other reasons (specify):

---

[1] Can be any other risk group that is surveyed.
[2] This period can be longer or shorter, depending on the findings from the formative research. This question also needs to be phrased according to the eligibility criteria of the survey.
[3] Or any other exclusion criteria relevant for the group that is surveyed.
[4] If that is the lower age limit for the survey.

Appendix 3.6

Non-eligibility form

Instructions. This form is completed by a screener whose task is to confirm whether a participant meets the inclusion (eligibility) criteria. If a participant does not meet eligibility criteria, this form needs to be filled out.

Reasons for not meeting eligibility criteria:

1. Person is not an MSM[1]

2. Person is an MSM but has not had anal sex in the past year

3. Under 18 years

4. Person is an MSM but does not study, work or live in city *XX*

5. Other (specif):

Complete this form for each person who comes to the site and does NOT meet the inclusion criteria to participate in the study.

NUMBER	COUPON NUMBER	DATE	REASON FOR NON-ELIGIBILITY (Write the code from the list above)	IF OTHER, SPECIFY	SCREENER SIGNATURE
1					
2					
3					
4					
5					
6					
7					
8					
9					
10					

---

[1] Important. The non-eligibility form should be adapted according to the eligibility criteria of the survey.

Appendix 3.7

Refuse to participate form

Instructions. This form is completed for each person who refuses to participate after a screener has confirmed that he/she meets the inclusion criteria. Participants can refuse to participate at any stage of the study, and the reasons for refusal need to be written in the form below.

Reasons for refusal

1. Did not want to sign consent
2. Did not want to answer questions
3. Fear of being identified
4. No time[1]
5. Did not want to give blood (or other specimens)
6. Other (specify):

NUMBER	COUPON NUMBER (Take away the coupon and file it in an envelope)	DATE	REASON FOR REFUSAL (Write the code from the list above)	IF OTHER, SPECIFY	SCREENER SIGNATURE
1					
2					
3					
4					
5					
6					
7					
8					
9					
10					

---

[1] Ask a participant whether he is willing to come back later. If yes, put his coupon in an envelope and try to make an appointment for the interview.

Appendix 3.8

Coupon rejecters form (non-response form)

*Instructions.*This form is used to estimate the extent of non-response in RDS by asking those who were distributing coupons how many people refused to accept a coupon. The form is filled out when those who participated come to the site to pick up a secondary incentive.

Survey ID code of a participant: _______________________________________

Coupon identification number: _______________________________________

Name of interviewer:____

Date of interview: ____

1. Is this the first time you have been here to collect compensation?
    Yes_____________   No _____________
    (If yes, continue. If no, answer questions for the period of time between when a participant was last here and filled out this same questionnaire and now)

2. How many coupons did you give out? _________________
    (Between the last time you came here to receive a secondary incentive and now)

3. How many people refused to accept coupons? _________
    (If zero, do not complete the rest of this questionnaire. If > zero, continue)

Complete the form below by asking the returning recruiter for the name of each person who refused to accept coupons. Read the questions.

QUESTIONS		PERSON 1	PERSON 2	PERSON 3	PERSON 4
1. What is your relationship to a person that you offered a coupon to?	A stranger, someone you met for the first time	1	1	1	1
	Someone you knew, but not closely	2	2	2	2
	A close friend, someone you knew very well	3	3	3	3
	A sex partner	4	4	4	4
	A family member or relative	5	5	5	5
2. How long have you known this person?	Less than 6 months	1	1	1	1
	6 months to 1 year	2	2	2	2
	1–2 years	3	3	3	3
	3–5 years	4	4	4	4
	More than 5 years	5	5	5	5
3. What do you think was the main reason given for refusing to accept a coupon? *(Do not read answers)*	Too busy	1	1	1	1
	Already had a coupon	2	2	2	2
	Not an MSM[1]	3	3	3	3
	Younger than 18 years	4	4	4	4
	Fear of being identified as an MSM	5	5	5	5
	Site is too far away	6	6	6	6
	Not interested	7	7	7	7
	Incentive is not worth the time	8	8	8	8
	Other (specify):	9	9	9	9

[1]   Or other member of the target population.

Appendix 3.9

Example of an information sheet for RDS participants of a study among MSM

Instructions. This sheet provides information about when and where participants can pick up their test results and how they should distribute coupons. This information sheet is explained and given to a participant by a coupon manager once a participant completes all steps of an RDS study.

HIV Testing and Counselling Centre

1 Palm Street, 21511 Sun City, Menaland

Tel: 03 483 0090

When and where can laboratory tests results be collected?

Test results can be collected *three weeks* after you participate in the survey (i.e. completed a questionnaire and gave specimens). Results can be collected from 2 pm to 3 pm from Sunday to Thursday at the same place as you gave specimens: the **HIV Testing and Counselling Centre, 1 Palm Street, 21511 Sun City**. The code that you have on this sheet is very important for you to keep as you will use it to collect your test results.

When and where can secondary incentives be collected?

You can collect a secondary incentive of 50 cents when a person to whom you gave a coupon is included in the survey. That means that your recruit needs to come to the site, fill out a questionnaire and give specimens for testing. After he completes all the steps in the study, you will be eligible for the secondary incentive. Please tell your peers to whom you give coupons that they need to come to the site before the date that is written on the coupon, which is two weeks from today. It is highly likely that you will be able to collect your secondary incentive when you come to pick up your test results.

Giving out coupons

Please give the coupons to your peers who are men who have sex with men, are aged 18 and over and have had anal sex in the past 12 months. It is written clearly on the coupon when they need to come to the HIV Testing and Counselling Centre in order to be included in the survey. In order to avoid waiting at the site, they can make an appointment at the following phone number: 03 483 0090. When you give them a coupon, please mention that:

- they will be tested for HIV and sexually transmitted infections for free
- the study is entirely confidential and anonymous
- participation in a study does not cause any risks to health
- those who participate will be reimbursed fully for the time lost and costs of transport.

What if someone refuses to accept a coupon?

If someone refuses to accept a coupon, please ask that person what the reasons for refusal are. Please try to remember this as it is important for the study. When you come back to the site, a staff member will ask you why people refused to accept coupons.

Thank you for participating in the study and distributing coupons!

Data collection forms used in HIV sentinel surveillance in ANC, TB and STI clinics

Appendix 3.10

Data collection form used in unlinked anonymous HIV surveillance in ANC clinics

NO.	QUESTIONS	CODING CATEGORIES
	Survey ID code	
	Clinic code	
	Patient ID number	
Q1	Date of patient visit	(dd/mm/yy) ___________|___________|___________|
Q2	Residence (town, village)	Urban 1 Peri-urban 2 Rural 3
Q3	Age (in years)	
Q4	Highest level of school completed	None 0 Primary 1 Secondary 2 Higher 3 Not known 9
Q5	Occupation	Farmer 1 Housewife 2 Labourer 3 Business 4 Police/military 5 Student 6 Professional 7 Not employed 8 Other 10 Not known 9
Q6	Total number of pregnancies, including this pregnancy	

Test results

<table>
<tr><td>HIV</td><td>Screening (initial) test date</td><td>(dd/mm/yy) ___________ | ___________ | ___________ |</td></tr>
<tr><td></td><td></td><td>Positive ☐ Negative ☐</td></tr>
<tr><td></td><td>Confirmatory test date</td><td>(dd/mm/yy) ___________ | ___________ | ___________ |</td></tr>
<tr><td></td><td></td><td>Positive ☐ Negative ☐</td></tr>
<tr><td>SYPHILIS</td><td>Screening (initial) test date</td><td>(dd/mm/yy) ___________ | ___________ | ___________ |</td></tr>
<tr><td></td><td></td><td>Positive ☐ Negative ☐</td></tr>
</table>

Appendix 3.11

Data collection form used in unlinked anonymous HIV surveillance in TB clinics

NO.	QUESTIONS	CODING CATEGORIES
	Survey ID code	
	Clinic code	
	Patient ID number	
Q1	Date of patient visit	(dd/mm/yy) ______|______|______
Q2	Residence (town, village)	Urban 1 Peri-urban 2 Rural 3
Q3	Age (in years)	
Q4	Sex	Male 1 Female 2
Q5	Highest level of school completed	None 0 Primary 1 Secondary 2 Higher 3 Not known 9
Q6	Occupation	Farmer 1 Housewife 2 Labourer 3 Business 4 Police/military 5 Student 6 Professional 7 Not employed 8 Other 10 Not known 9
Q7	Clinical presentation of tuberculosis	Pulmonary ☐ Extrapulmonary ☐ If pulmonary: Sputum smear positive ☐ Sputum smear negative ☐

Test results

<table>
<tr><td>HIV</td><td>Screening (initial) test date</td><td>(dd/mm/yy) ___ / ___ / ___</td></tr>
<tr><td></td><td></td><td>Positive ☐ Negative ☐</td></tr>
<tr><td></td><td>Confirmatory test date</td><td>(dd/mm/yy) ___ / ___ / ___</td></tr>
<tr><td></td><td></td><td>Positive ☐ Negative ☐</td></tr>
</table>

Appendix 3.12

Data collection form used in unlinked anonymous HIV surveillance in STI clinics

NO.	QUESTIONS	CODING CATEGORIES
	Survey ID code	
	Clinic code	
	Patient ID number	
Q1	Date of patient visit	(dd/mm/yy) ______ | ______ | ______ |
Q2	Residence (town, village)	Urban 1 Peri-urban 2 Rural 3
Q3	Age (in years)	
Q4	Sex	Male 1 Female 2
Q5	Highest level of school completed	None 0 Primary 1 Secondary 2 Higher 3 Not known 9
Q6	Occupation	Farmer 1 Housewife 2 Labourer 3 Business 4 Police/military 5 Student 6 Professional 7 Not employed 8 Other 10 Not known 9
Q7	Number of partners in past three months	
Q8	Sex of partners in past three months	Only women 1 Only men 2 Both men and women 3 Not known 9
Q9	Injection drug use in past three months	Yes 1 No 2 Not known 9
Q10	Paid for sex or sold sex in past six months	Yes 1 No 2 Not known 9

Test results

PRESENCE OF SYMPTOMS AND/OR STI DIAGNOSED		DATE AND TYPE OF TEST		
Patient presented with		Urethral discharge 1 Genital ulcer 2 Vaginal discharge 3 Lower abdominal pain 4 Inguinal bubo 5 Asymptomatic (no discharge and/or dysuria) 6		
HIV	Screening (initial) test date	(dd/mm/yy) ______ | ______ | ______ |		
		Positive ☐ Negative ☐		
	Confirmatory test date	(dd/mm/yy) ______ | ______ | ______ |		
		Positive ☐ Negative ☐		
Syphilis	Screening test date (RPR, VDRL)	(dd/mm/yy) ______ | ______ | ______ |		
		Positive ☐ Negative ☐ Not tested ☐		
	Confirmatory test date	(dd/mm/yy) ______ | ______ | ______ |		
		Positive ☐ Negative ☐ Not tested ☐		
Gonorrhoea	Type of test	Positive ☐ Negative ☐ Not tested ☐		
Chlamydia	Type of test	Positive ☐ Negative ☐ Not tested ☐		
Herpes	Type of test	Positive ☐ Negative ☐ Not tested ☐		
Chancroid	Type of test	Positive ☐ Negative ☐ Not tested ☐		

References

1   Hulley SB, Cummings SR, Browner WS, Grady D, Hearst N, Newman TB. *Designing clinical research. An epidemiological approach,* 2nd ed. Philadelphia, Lippincott, Williams and Wilkins, 2001.

2   Swai RO, Somi GR, Matee MI, Killewo J, Lyamuya EF, Kwesigabo G, Tulli T, Kabalimu T, Ng'ang'a L, Isingo R, Ndayongeje J. Surveillance of HIV and syphilis infections among antenatal clinic attendees in Tanzania—2003/2004. *BMC public health*, 2006, 6:91.

3   Kerr-Pontes LR, Gondin R, Mota RS, Martins TA, Wypij D. Self-reported sexual behaviour and HIV risk taking among men who have sex with men in Fortaleza, Brazil. *AIDS*, 1999, 13:709–17.

4   Deaux E, Callaghan JW. Key informant versus self-report estimates of health behavior. *Evaluation review*, 1985, 9:365–8.

5   Waters JK, Biernacki P. Targeted sampling: options for the study of hidden populations. *Social problems*, 1989, 36(4):416–30.

6   *Guidelines for appropriate evaluations of HIV testing technologies in Africa. Based on a workgroup meeting in Harare.* Atlanta, Georgia, WHO Regional Office for Africa/Centers for Disease Control and Prevention, 2002.

7   Grassly NC, Morgan M, Walker N, Garnett G, Stanecki KA, Stover J, Brown T, Ghys PD. Uncertainty in estimates of HIV/AIDS: the estimation and application of plausibility bounds. *Sexually transmitted infections*, 2004, 80(suppl. 1):i31–i38.

8   Kwesigabo G, Killewo JZ, Urassa W, Mbena E, Mhalu F, Lugalla JL, Godoy C, Biberfeld G, Emmelin M, Wall S, Sandstrom A. Monitoring of HIV-1 infection prevalence and trends in the general population: 9 years experience from the Kagera region of Tanzania. *Journal of acquired immune deficiency syndromes*, 2000, 23(5):410–17

9   *Responding to surveillance: methods and software to produce HIV/AIDS estimates in the era of population-based prevalence surveys. Technical recommendations.* Geneva, UNAIDS, 2004. Report of a meeting of the UNAIDS Reference Group for "Estimates, Modelling and Projections".

10 Saphonn V, Hor BL, Ly SP, Chhuon S, Saidel T, Dteles R. How well do antenatal clinic (ANC) attendees represent the general population? A comparison of HIV prevalence from ANC sentinel surveillance sites with a population-based survey of women 15–49 in Cambodia. *Journal of epidemiology*, 2002, 31:449–55.

11 Fylkesnes K, Ndhlovu Z, Kasumba K, Musonda RM. Sichone M. Studying dynamics of the HIV epidemic: population-based data compared with sentinel surveillance in Zambia. *AIDS*, 1998, 12:1227–34.

12 Boerma JT, Ghys PD, Walker N. Estimates of HIV-1 prevalence from national population-based surveys as a new gold standard. *Lancet*, 2003, 362(9399):1929–31.

13 Lemeshow S, Hosmer DW, Janelle K, Lwanga SK. *Adequacy of sample size in health studies*. New York, John Wiley & Sons, 1990.

14 *Behavioral surveillance surveys. Guidelines for repeated behavioral surveys in populations at risk of HIV.* Durham, North Carolina, Family Health International, 2000.

15 Van Griensven F, Thanprasertsuk S, Jommaroeng R, Mansergh G, Naorat S, Jenkins RA, Ungchusak K, Phanuphak P, Tappero JW. Bangkok MSM Study Group. Evidence of a previously undocumented epidemic of HIV infection among men who have sex with men in Bangkok, Thailand. *AIDS*, 2005, 19(5):521–6.

16 Muhib FB, Lin LS, Stueve A, Miller RL, Ford WL, Johnson WD, Smith PJ. Community intervention trial for youth study team. A venue-based method for sampling hard-to-reach populations. *Public health reports*, 2001, 116(suppl. 1):216–22.

17 Stueve A, O'Donnell LN, Duran R, San Doval A, Blome J. Time-space sampling in minority communities: results with young Latino men who have sex with men. *American journal of public health,* 2001; 91(6):922–6.

18 Spreen M, Zwaagstra R. Personal network sampling, outdegree analysis and multilevel analysis: introducing the network concept in studies of hidden populations. *International sociology*, 1994, 9:475–91.

19 Broadhead RS, Heckathorn DD. AIDS prevention outreach among injection drug users: agency problems and new approaches. *Social problems*, 1994, 41:473–95.

20 Broadhead RS, Heckathorn DD, Grund JPC, Stern LS, Anthony DL. Drug users versus outreach workers in combating AIDS: preliminary results of a peer-driven intervention. *Journal of drug issues*, 1995, 25(3):531–64.

21 Ramirez-Valles J, Heckathorn DD, Vazquez R, Diaz RM, Campbell RT. From networks to populations: the development and application of respondent-driven sampling among IDUs and Latino gay men. *AIDS and behaviour*, 2005, 9(4):387–402.

22 Heckathorn D. Respondent-driven sampling: a new approach to the study of hidden populations. *Social problems*, 1997, 44(2):174–99.

23 Heckathorn D. Respondent-driven sampling II: deriving valid population estimates from chain-referral samples of hidden populations. *Social problems*, 2002. 49(1):11–34.

24 Johnston LG. *Conducting respondent driven sampling (RDS) studies in diverse settings: a manual for planning RDS studies.* Atlanta, Georgia, Centers for Disease Control, 2007.

25 Kirkwood BR, Sterne JAC. *Medical statistics*, 2nd ed. Oxford, Blackwell Science, 2003.

26 UNAIDS/WHO Working Group on Global HIV/AIDS and STI surveillance. *Guidelines for measuring national HIV prevalence in population based surveys.* Geneva, UNAIDS/WHO, 2005.

27 *Estimating the size of populations at risk for HIV.* Arlington, Virginia, Family Health International, 2003.

Part 4

Collecting information from participants in surveillance

4.1

Introduction

Part 4 describes principles of collecting biological and behavioural data in HIV surveillance activities. Chapter 4.2 addresses standardized case definitions of HIV infection, advanced HIV disease and AIDS in surveillance activities. Examples of testing modalities used in HIV surveillance are described in chapter 4.3. Practical issues related to blood sample collection are addressed in chapter 4.4. Chapter 4.5 describes behavioural data collection with a focus on levels and trends in sexual and drug-taking behaviour linked to HIV transmission; attitudes, beliefs and knowledge about HIV; and other indicators used to track the epidemic, its response, and its impact. Chapter 4.6 provides practical guidance on the implementation of surveillance surveys, and chapter 4.7 highlights ethical considerations in HIV surveillance.

4.2

Biological data collection

4.2.1 Case definitions of HIV infection and AIDS and case-based surveillance systems

A case definition is the set of clinical and/or laboratory criteria that a patient must have in order to be counted as an occurrence of an infection or disease for surveillance purposes. Case-based surveillance is the systematic recording of all cases diagnosed among persons seeking medical services and reported by health care providers to public health officials. Such systems form a core activity of HIV surveillance systems worldwide in all stages of the epidemic. However, in and of themselves they provide an incomplete picture of the HIV epidemic as many persons with HIV do not seek medical care for many years, there can be severe underdiagnosis of cases, underreporting of diagnosed cases and potential duplication of known cases.

The basic analysis of HIV and AIDS case surveillance data involves the absolute count of cases overall and by person, place and time [1]. Case surveillance data can provide a sense of the major modes of transmission present in a country or region; the relative burden of disease by age, sex and geography; and changes in these factors over time. These data elements (age, sex and geography, at minimum) are collected with each new case reported. Countries vary according to whether cases are reported individually with the name and other identifying information on each case, by a non-identifying code assigned to each case, or aggregated by reporting site, district or region without being able to distinguish individual cases, as is done in integrated disease surveillance systems. With individual case reporting, the stage of disease at the time of initial diagnosis is ideally reported with each new case.

During 2004–06, WHO led a consensus process to revise the HIV case definition for surveillance and treatment and to harmonize this definition with the clinical and immunological classification of HIV [2]. The aim of this revision was to make HIV case reporting more applicable to clinical management and treatment, particularly for countries with limited laboratory capacity, and with a view to scaling up access to HIV treatment globally. HIV-related disease and immunological classification for adults and children[1] are described in a four-stage system presented in Tables 4.1 and 4.2 below.

---

[1] For the purposes of HIV case definitions for reporting and surveillance, children are defined as younger than 15 years.

Table 4.1 WHO clinical classification of established HIV infection

HIV-associated symptomatology	WHO clinical stage
Asymptomatic	1
Mild symptoms	2
Advanced symptoms	3
Severe symptoms	4

The events used to categorize HIV disease are divided into those for which a presumptive clinical diagnosis can be made (i.e. where syndromes or conditions can be diagnosed clinically or with basic laboratory tests) and those which require a definitive diagnosis (etiologically described conditions requiring more sophisticated laboratory tests). Table 4.1 outlines the clinical staging of HIV infection (asymptomatic, mildly symptomatic, advanced symptoms and severely symptomatic).

The standard assessment of immunological status of the HIV-infected child or adult is measured by the absolute number (/mm^3) or percentage of CD4 cells with the revised WHO immunological classification system by age presented in Table 4.2 below. The CD4 values have prognostic purposes and are used to estimate the need for antiretroviral therapy (ART)[1]. In children less than 5 years of age, the absolute CD4 count varies within an individual child more than the percentage CD4 and therefore the percentage CD4 is used for classification in younger children.

Table 4.2 WHO immunological classification of established HIV infection

HIV-associated immunodeficiency	Age-related CD4 values			
	≤11 months (% CD4)	12–35 months (% CD4)	36–59 months (% CD4)	≥5 years (absolute number per mm^3 or % CD4)
None or not significant	>35	>30	>25	>500
Mild	30–35	25–30	20–25	350–499
Advanced	25–29	20–24	15–29	200–349
Severe	<25	<20	<15	<200 or <15%

---

[1] The pathogenesis of HIV infection is largely attributable to the decrease in the number of CD4 lymphocytes. Progressive depletion of CD4 T-cells is associated with progression of HIV, with increased likelihood of opportunistic infections and other clinical events associated with HIV.

WHO recommends that national programmes standardize and review their HIV and AIDS case definitions in the light of these revisions. For further information on the revised case definitions and their impact on HIV surveillance, the reader is referred to the document[1] *WHO case definitions of HIV for surveillance, and revised clinical staging and immunological classification of HIV related disease in adults and children.* Geneva, WHO, 2006. Available at http://www.who.int/hiv/pub/guidelines/who%20hiv%20Staging.pdf.

Appendixes 4.1 and 4.2 provide examples of HIV and AIDS case reporting forms for adults, adolescents and children.

---

[1] In this publication, there are also a description of WHO clinical staging of HIV for adults, adolescents and children and presumptive and definitive criteria for recognizing HIV-related clinical events.

4.3

Laboratory testing technologies and strategies for surveillance

4.3.1　HIV antibody testing

The most common means to detect the presence of HIV infection, to measure HIV prevalence in populations and screen persons for definitive diagnosis and clinical staging is the HIV antibody test. Since the mid 1980s, when HIV testing first became available, there has been a proliferation of assays to detect HIV antibodies. Tests have progressively increased their sensitivity and specificity, their range of different subtypes they detect (including HIV-1 and HIV-2), the specimen type used (e.g. blood collection, finger stick, oral secretions, urine) and their modality (e.g. conducted in laboratories in batches or singly by rapid, point-of-use tests). Most are based on variations of the enzyme-linked immunoassay (EIA) method, which detects the presence of HIV-specific antibodies. Other assays include the detection of antigens in the specimens themselves.

A single HIV-positive EIA or rapid test result usually does not make a definitive diagnosis for clinical purposes. Rather, confirmation of a case relies on additional testing, either with a second or third different EIA or rapid test or with a western blot test. A complete description of all HIV antibody tests and the algorithms for screening and confirmation is beyond the scope of these guidelines. Moreover, the assays available and approved for use depend on each country's specific guidelines, regulations and systems of internal and external quality control. Readers are therefore referred to their national reference laboratory for the currently recommended HIV antibody testing assays and algorithms. The table below provides a comparison of the conventional EIA versus rapid test modalities of HIV antibody testing for HIV surveillance applications.

4.3.2 Comparison of HIV testing technologies: enzyme immunoassays and rapid tests

HIV testing technology	Specimen	Advantages	Limitations	Cost (US$)	Complexity (from 1 [simple] to 4 [highly complex])
Conventional enzyme immunoassays (EIA)	Serum Plasma Dried blood spots Oral fluid	Can be batched: good for 90 specimens at a time Can be automated Quality control; easier to control Highly sensitive, reduces window period if fourth-generation EIA	Requires skilled, trained technicians to perform testing and calculate results Can take two hours or longer depending on batching Requires special equipment Requires maintenance of equipment Kits require refrigeration	0.5–1	4
Rapid test	Serum Plasma Whole blood Oral fluid	Requires minimal equipment and reagents Can be performed outside a laboratory (on-site testing) Test results easy to interpret Results in 30 minutes or less Most kits can be stored at up to 30 °C	Less efficient for large numbers of specimens Positive and negative control specimens often not included in the kit	0.5–4	For tests based on: immunochromatography 1 dipstick and flow-through devices 1–2 agglutination 2–3

4.3.3 Laboratory methods for HIV incidence surveillance

An assay that can determine if a person has recent or long-term infection would have enormous value to HIV surveillance. Distinguishing recent from longer-standing infection enables characterizing where HIV transmission is happening at present, therefore directing HIV prevention efforts to where they are needed most. However, detection of recent HIV infection has been an ongoing challenge in HIV surveillance. At present, several tests and testing algorithms for recent infection detection and incidence estimation are under development.

The sequence of immunological events starting from the first few days through first several months of infection provides opportunities to identify persons with recent infection [5, 8]. The basic approach is to apply an assay that is sensitive to detecting infection in early stages and a second assay that detects infection in later stages and using the known timing of these events to classify the duration of infection. Knowing the timing of the events also permits estimation of HIV incidence as a rate. When based on certain serological tests, this overall approach is sometimes referred to as serological testing algorithm for recent HIV-1 seroconversion or STARHS. A recent review of the assays for recent infection detection and HIV incidence estimation can be found at http://www. eurosurveillance.org/ViewArticle.aspx?Articleid=18966). The following describes the principles behind some of the more common HIV incidence assays and algorithms used in surveillance.

p24 antigen

HIV p24 antigen is a viral protein that appears in the serum of HIV-infected persons at about 14 days after actual infection and approximately one week before the appearance of HIV antibodies. Thus, a person testing HIV antibody–negative yet p24 antigen–positive is presumed to be very recently infected. This narrow period of detecting recent infection makes the p24/HIV-antibody testing algorithm inefficient outside of settings where programmes are testing very large numbers of specimens (e.g. blood banks) or very high rates of recent infection (e.g. STI clinics).

HIV RNA and DNA

HIV RNA and DNA (nucleic acids) appear about 7–10 days after infection and a few weeks before the appearance of HIV antibodies. Therefore, like p24 antigen, there is a short period when someone recently infected is nucleic acid–positive and HIV antibody–negative. Pooling of specimens to test for HIV nucleic acid reduces considerably the costs of testing individually. In cases where a pool tests positive, the specimens comprising the pool then are tested in order to determine which individual specimens are HIV-positive. These methods are not often used for routine surveillance but are common in blood banks to ensure the safety of donated blood. Of note, the early period of HIV infection where nucleic acid is detectable is thought to be highly contagious, and therefore prevention efforts targeting this period may have benefit in controlling the epidemic.

Less sensitive assay

The less sensitive or detuned assay determines early infection based on the slow rise in HIV antibody titre over the first six months of infection. A sensitive EIA will detect antibodies approximately 21 days after infection, while the less sensitive (detuned) EIA detects antibodies approximately 170 days after infection. Thus, a blood specimen reactive on a sensitive EIA but non-reactive on the less sensitive EIA is presumed to be from a person infected within the previous six months. To date, STARHS has been generally calibrated and applied to type B strains of HIV-1, and the sensitivity and specificity for detecting recent infection are only in the range of 80%–85% [9, 10].

BED assay

The BED test is based on the slow rise in the proportion of antibodies specific to gp41, a glycoprotein involved in helping HIV enter human cells, in relation to total antibodies.

The BED assay was constructed of antigens from HIV types B, E and D and has cross-reactivity with many other strains. The BED assay classifies persons in the first 153 days after seroconversion or later. Due to its ability to react to many strains of HIV the BED assay has been applied to HIV surveillance in many settings. However, there have been many concerns in the performance and validation of the BED assay. Comparisons of BED assay–derived measures of HIV incidence with other methods suggest that the BED overestimates incidence by falsely classifying persons with long-standing infection as recent [11]. In addition to a small population of persons who do not appear to evolve high gp41 antibody responses, other factors affecting the estimate of incidence include antiretroviral therapy, severe immunosuppression, high levels of total antibody and HIV-2. While BED assay is not yet recommended for routine surveillance, the US Centers for Disease Control and Prevention have issued interim recommendations for its use for incidence estimations [12].

4.3.4   Laboratory tests for detection of hepatitis

Groups at high risk of parenterally acquiring HIV, such as IDU, also have increased risk of other bloodborne infections such as hepatitis B and C. In some settings, serological testing for these infections may signal risk for HIV. In addition, screening for these diseases can have public health benefits in itself as these infections are a major source of morbidity and mortality. When incorporated into surveillance activities, appropriate referral for care and vaccination for hepatitis B should be in place for survey participants.

Hepatitis B

Hepatitis B in much of the world is acquired in early childhood and is therefore not a consistent marker for injection drug use or sexual risk in adults. Moreover, there has been a scale-up of hepatitis B vaccination worldwide. Several tests are required to determine the hepatitis B infection status of an individual [14]:

- antibody to hepatitis B core protein (anti-HBc) is a marker of past or ongoing infection, appearing at the onset of symptoms in acute hepatitis B and persisting for life
- antibody to hepatitis B surface protein (anti-HBs) is associated with past naturally occurring infection or prior vaccination; it is generally interpreted as indicating recovery from and immunity to hepatitis B virus
- hepatitis B surface antigen (HBsAg) is a marker of ongoing hepatitis B virus replication and can be due to either acute or chronic infection.

Hepatitis C

Hepatitis C spreads rapidly through populations of IDU who share needles and is therefore a fairly reliable marker for injection risk of HIV. Hepatitis C is typically measured through EIA. Although EIA can detect more than 95% of chronically infected patients, they can detect only 50% to 70% of acute infections. For this reason, a recombinant immunoblot assay (RIBA) or hepatitis C RNA assay is used as confirmatory test for hepatitis C infection [15].

4.4

Biological sample collection procedures and results return

When planning the biological component of surveillance surveys, several issues must be addressed, such as where biological specimens can be collected (health care settings or other sites such as those run by nongovernmental organizations), who can collect them (trained lay people, registered nurses, medical technicians, doctors), and what type of specimen will be collected (whole blood by venipuncture or fingerprick, oral fluid, urine). The procedures of specimen transport and testing will depend on the proximity of the site where sampling is done to the laboratory and the testing algorithms that are in place in a country. Specimens and data collection forms can be transported during the supervisory visits to the laboratory. Receipt forms need to document the number of samples transported and handed over to the laboratory.

Each biological specimen should be labelled with a unique survey code, which is the same code that is assigned to the questionnaire and other data collection forms, in order to enable linking of biological and behavioural data. Storage of specimens depends on the type of specimen. If serum samples will be tested for HIV more than three days after collection, they should be stored at −20 °C. For longer-term storage (e.g. years), serum should be frozen at −70 °C. Dried blood spots can be stored at room temperature in storage bags for up to 30 days or at 4 °C for up to 90 days. For longer storage, they should be kept at −20 °C [16]. During transport, serum specimens should be packed in coolers.

In community-based surveillance surveys, biological specimens should be collected at the same site as the interview, and the site should therefore have a private area for sample collection. In linked anonymous HIV surveys, where results are given back, participants should receive pre- and post-test counselling. It is best if results are provided at the site where testing was done. If that is not feasible, results can be collected from a nearby collaborating VCT centre. In the event that results are not possible or feasible to return, every measure possible must be taken to ensure that persons who wish to know their HIV status are able to do so. This may include vouchers for free HIV testing and counselling at the nearest centre or the parallel provision of mobile VCT alongside the survey. Provision of such services will increase the cost and complexity of survey operations, but will also bring more benefit to individuals who participate in the survey and the wider community. Participants with symptoms or signs suggestive of HIV or other STI should receive treatment based on national or WHO guidelines. In situations where treatment cannot be provided on site, referrals should be made to nearby clinics for free treatment. Study participants should be provided with health education materials on HIV and STI (leaflets, informational brochures) and with condoms.

Readers are referred to more comprehensive documents regarding sample transport and storage, such as:

- *Guidelines for using HIV testing technologies in surveillance: selection, evaluation and implementation – 2009 update.* Geneva, WHO, 2010. Available at http://www.who.int/hiv/pub/surveillance/hiv_testing_technologies_surveillance_.pdf
- *Guidelines for appropriate evaluations of HIV testing technologies in Africa. Based on a workgroup meeting in Harare.* Atlanta, Georgia, WHO Regional Office for Africa/Centers for Disease Control. Available at http://www.who.int/diagnostics_laboratory/publications/EN_hivEval_Guide.pdf.

4.5

Behavioural data collection

4.5.1 The role of behavioural surveillance surveys in HIV surveillance

Behavioural surveillance is the ongoing systematic collection, analysis and interpretation of behavioural data relevant to understanding trends in the transmission of infection [17]. Data on sexual and drug-using behaviour assess the potential for an HIV epidemic to emerge or spread and thus serve as an early warning system. Other roles of behavioural surveillance are to inform the design of interventions by identifying which population subgroups are at risk for HIV and which specific behaviour prevention programmes need to target; to assess the level of knowledge about the modes of HIV and STI transmission and the ways for people to protect themselves; to determine the use of various means of protection; and to help set priorities for interventions. Behavioural surveillance cannot be used on its own to evaluate the effectiveness of specific programmes or interventions, but can be used to assess whether prevention efforts within a community are reaching important population segments and meeting the local and national objectives of HIV prevention.

Behavioural surveillance surveys systematically monitor levels and trends in HIV-related risk behaviour across different populations and over time in key target groups. In this type of surveillance, the design is a series of repeated cross-sectional surveys conducted at regular intervals coordinated on a national or regional scale. Increasingly, collection of behavioural and biological data is done simultaneously, with both sets of data being collected from the same participants (i.e. integrated bio-behavioural surveillance or IBBS). This multiple data collection enhances the use and explanatory power of surveillance surveys by directly linking the behavioural causes associated with the biological outcome of infection.

4.5.2 Behavioural data collection questionnaires

Behavioural data are collected by administering standardized questionnaires, which for HIV surveillance include measures of:

- sociodemographic characteristics
- drug and injection drug use
- sexual behaviour
- knowledge of modes of HIV and STI transmission and sources of knowledge
- attitudes towards HIV and stigma and discrimination towards people living with HIV

- perception of the risk of HIV
- the use of prevention and other HIV-related services, including contact with drug treatment and harm reduction services.

Of note, it should be anticipated that groups at risk for HIV are often exposed through multiple mechanisms. For example, female sex workers might also inject drugs.

Questionnaires can be administered many ways, including the following.

- Face-to-face interviews. An interviewer reads questions to the respondent and records answers on the questionnaire. This has the advantage of being consistent for literate and illiterate participants. Another advantage is that complicated questions can be explained and clarified by an interviewer, which may not possible if the questionnaire is self-administered. A disadvantage is that respondents might not provide accurate answers on sensitive questions when appearing in front of the interviewer.
- Self-administered questionnaire. Respondents are given a questionnaire which they read and complete themselves.
- Computer-assisted interviewing. Similar to self-administered, but respondents read and complete the questionnaire using a computer. This method further protects anonymity and confidentiality, but requires computers on site or portable computers in the field. Research suggests that computer-assisted interviewing may produce more valid reports of sensitive behaviour than face-to-face interviews [18, 19].

Formative research during the pre-surveillance assessment provides information on how to phrase the questions and what terminology to use. Before a questionnaire is finalized, it should be pre-tested with members of the target population to ensure the clarity of questions, the appropriate flow of questions and to assess the time needed to complete the questionnaire. An interviewer guide should be also available for staff to ensure that everyone is following the same procedures when interviewing. Pre-testing of a questionnaire is done during preparation for the surveillance survey; the goals of pre-testing are:

- to estimate how long it takes to administer the questionnaire
- to determine the appropriate sequencing of sections and questions
- to identify whether the wording is clear and understandable to those being interviewed
- to assess whether some issues require clarification during the interview; if so, they have to be explained either by an interviewer or in writing
- to assess the skills of interviewing staff.

Pre-testing a questionnaire identifies potential sources of error that affect the quality of results. For example, ambiguous wording, too many questions, time-frame too long for measuring relatively common behaviour so respondents have difficulty remembering, or time-frame too short for measuring rare behaviour (i.e. asking participants to report on behaviour in the past six months when on average individuals only engage in that behaviour a few times or even once a year). Many errors from discomfort can be reduced by placing sensitive questions towards the end of the questionnaire, starting with general questions and moving towards specific ones, making sure questions are non-judgemental, using wording that is as simple and clear as possible and avoiding abbreviations and scientific jargon.

Ideally, questionnaires should be developed locally in the local language and context. However, the trade-off is that questions may not be comparable across or within countries. Therefore, there is great advantage in using, translating and pilot-testing standardized questionnaires that have been already piloted in similar settings. Further information on behavioural data collection and standardized questionnaires for female sex workers, men who have sex with men, injection drug users, unmarried young people and adults are available from:

- *Behavioral surveillance surveys. Guidelines for repeated behavioral surveys in populations at risk of HIV*. Durham, North Carolina, Family Health International, 2000. Available at http://www.fhi.org/en/HIVAIDS/pub/guide/bssguidelines.htm.

Moreover, the current era has seen the need for internationally standardized indicators to monitor global progress in fighting the epidemic. For example, the United Nations General Assembly Special Session on HIV (UNGASS), UNAIDS and WHO have developed a standardized set of indicators requested of all countries. Many of the indicators are derived from HIV surveillance behavioural surveys and are specifically defined with respect to time-frames and content. Examples of indicators and corresponding variables for inclusion in behavioural surveys are presented in Table 4.3 below. Details on the specific construction of the UNGASS indicators can be found at http://data.unaids.org/pub/Manual/2007/20070411_ungass_core_indicators_manual_en.pdf

Other publications that contain behavioural and programme-related indicators are available at http://www.who.int/hiv/pub/me/en/.

---

[1] In addition to HIV prevalence, surveys can include measurement of HIV incidence as this allows the estimation of recent transmission and provides better estimates of programme effectiveness. STI prevalence can also serve as an impact indicator.

Table 4.3 Programme indicators and corresponding variables for inclusion in behavioural surveys

	Indicator	**Variables for inclusion in behavioural surveys**
Injection drug users	Percentage of IDU reporting the use of sterile injecting equipment the last time they injected (UNGASS)	use of sterile injecting equipment the last time the respondent injected drugs
		having injected in the past month
	Frequency of injection	number of injections per week
		having injected drugs in the past month
	Percentage of IDU reporting the use of a condom the last time they had sexual intercourse (UNGASS)	use of a condom the most recent time the respondent had sex
		having had sexual intercourse in the past month
Sex workers	Percentage of sex workers reporting the use of a condom the most recent time they had sexual intercourse (UNGASS)	use of a condom the most recent time the respondent had sex
		having had sexual intercourse in the past month
	Number and type of sexual partners	number of clients in the past month
		number of regular non-client sexual partners (spouse or other) in the past month
Men who have sex with men	Percentage of MSM reporting the use of a condom the most recent time they had sexual intercourse (UNGASS)	use of a condom the most recent time the respondent had anal sex
		having had sexual intercourse in the past month
	Number and type of sexual partners	number of sexual partners in the past month
		number of paid sexual partners in the past month

4.6

Ensuring quality in surveillance: fieldwork and quality assurance

Two activities to ensure that surveillance surveys are of high quality entail monitoring the fieldwork and laboratory quality assurance. Laboratory quality assurance is not described in this document, but can be found at http://www.who.int/diagnostics_laboratory/ quality/en/. Information on quality control in molecular diagnostics can be found at http://www.qcmd.org/Index2.htm.

With respect to fieldwork, the following general measures will help ensure higher-quality data collection:

- employing experienced people and training them adequately
- clearly defining the roles and responsibilities of staff and providing regular supervision
- ensuring appropriate payment of staff
- employing an efficient study manager
- organizing daily follow-up and at least weekly meetings to discuss progress in data collection
- documenting difficulties encountered during any stage of data collection and brainstorming with the team to find solutions.

Supervision includes monitoring the quality of the entire process of behavioural and biological data collection. Supervisors have a vital role in ensuring that the survey is being run as planned.

All sites should be visited shortly before surveillance starts and as soon as possible after it starts. Supervisors need to regularly visit the study sites during data collection. The frequency of visits will depend on the types of data collected and overall capacities to adequately carry out data collection. The frequency of supervisory visits will depend on the design of the survey and needs to be discussed with staff during preparations for the survey.

Supervisors check at each visit whether all survey documentation and specimen storage and transport are managed according to the protocol, making sure that:

- all survey forms are properly filled out
- all questionnaires and test tubes are coded according to protocol

- there are sufficient supplies of laboratory materials, test kits and data collection forms
- storage of specimens is appropriate
- problems during data collection are addressed in a timely manner
- any necessary logistic arrangements for the team are made
- staff are motivated and attentive to problems
- participants are treated with respect, and there is a mechanism in place for receiving and resolving complaints
- if some questions are consistently not properly answered, discuss this with interviewers and provide additional clarification to participants
- supervisors should be present occasionally during data collection to observe data collection practices.

When doing community-based surveys, field coordinators/supervisors should be available for consultation with interviewers at any time. They need to check every questionnaire either every day when field staff finish data collection, or if this is not feasible, then every second or third day of data collection. It is also helpful for supervisors to periodically sit in on a surveillance survey interview with each staff member. This will enable supervisors to give feedback and assess adherence to interviewer training/guidelines. The supervisor needs to assess the week's progress by checking:

- how many interviews were completed and at which sites (clusters) and (for cluster-based sampling) whether the target number of sites and interviews per site was met
- the number of completed interviews per interviewer
- the number of refusals per site
- transport of specimens
- any problems during fieldwork.

Supervision should be standardized using a checklist. The example on the next page refers to a checklist that can be used for clinic-based surveillance.

Site supervision checklist for clinic-based surveillance

Site name: _________________________   Site number: _________________________

Supervisor name: _________________________   Date: _________________________

Surveillance week no.: _________________________   Weekday: _________________________

Comments:

SAMPLING

Day with ANC care? ☐ Yes ☐ No: ____

Total no. women receiving ANC since surveillance started: _________________________

Total no. women sampled since surveillance started: _________________________

No. of women sampled on most recent ANC day: _________________________

Sampling consecutive? ☐ Yes ☐ No: ____

ANC staff present: ☐ Yes ☐ No: _________   Lab. tech. present: ☐ Yes ☐ No: _________

No. data forms: _________________________   No. blood samples: _________________________

Comments:

SUPPLIES: SUFFICIENT FOR NEXT FOUR WEEKS (100 PATIENTS)?

Vacutainers ☐ Yes ☐ No	Needles ☐ Yes ☐ No	Needle holders ☐ Yes ☐ No
Data forms ☐ Yes ☐ No	Labels ☐ Yes ☐ No	Alcohol/swabs ☐ Yes ☐ No
Tourniquets ☐ Yes ☐ No	Cryoboxes ☐ Yes ☐ No	Cryovials ☐ Yes ☐ No

Other materials needed:

Comments:

EQUIPMENT

Cryovials stored in fridge: ☐ Yes ☐ No: _________________________   Fridge temperature: _______

Fridge working uninterrupted since last visit? ☐ Yes ☐ No: _________________________

Centrifuge working? ☐ Yes ☐ No: ____

Comments:

SAMPLE TRANSPORT: ☐ Yes ☐ No: ____

No. samples taken: _________________________

Site staff name: _________________________

Site staff signature: _________________________

Comments:

4.7

Ethical issues in surveillance

Persons conducting HIV surveillance activities must adhere to the ethical principles guiding human subjects research, even when some such activities do not fall under the jurisdiction of research. An overview of ethical principles and guidelines can be found at http://ohsr.od.nih.gov/guidelines/belmont.html. This chapter deals with some of the ethical issues particular to HIV surveillance. Further information concerning ethical issues in surveillance can be found in the WHO publication *Ethical issues to be considered in second generation surveillance*, available at http://www.who.int/hiv/pub/epidemiology/en/sgs_ethical.pdf. In addition the Council for International Organizations of Medical Sciences (CIOMS) has recently (2007) published *International ethical guidelines for epidemiological studies*, available at http://www.cioms.ch/

4.7.1 Maximizing protection of study subjects

Surveillance is often conducted among people who are stigmatized and marginalized. In some countries certain sexual behaviour and drug use are punishable. Utmost caution should be taken in conducting surveillance activities among stigmatized populations in these situations. Every effort should be made to protect individuals from any and all adverse consequences or social/legal sanctions that may arise from other people knowing that they participated in an HIV survey or knowing their survey responses. There is also the possibility of discrimination if the results of any HIV or STI tests become known to others. Therefore, HIV surveillance surveys need to have the highest possible ethical standards and must ensure confidentiality and anonymity.

4.7.2 Ensuring confidentiality and anonymity

Whenever possible, surveillance activities should be conducted so that participation is totally anonymous as the most secure means of protecting participants from inadvertent disclosure of personal information. Anonymity in surveys may also increase participation and thus representation. If anonymity is not possible every effort must be made to ensure confidentiality.

Ways to ensure confidentiality include:

- not recording names or other identifiers anywhere. All study documents and specimens are labelled with only a non-identifying unique participant study number

- requesting informed consent verbally for all data collection (with the exception of unlinked anonymous surveillance)
- storing data safely in locked filing cabinets, in locked and guarded buildings and in password-protected computers
- training all surveillance staff on the importance of confidentiality.

Special epidemiological studies should be reviewed by ethical committees to be sure that ethical standards are respected and that measures to ensure confidentiality are strong.

At both the community and individual levels, creating an atmosphere of trust, ensuring confidentiality and emphasizing the importance of consent are crucial for involving vulnerable groups in surveillance activities.

4.7.3 Informed consent

Consent of adults

Informed consent is discussed with a potential participant at the very beginning of a survey. Before participants give informed consent, they must be told:

- the purpose of the survey
- a description of the procedures of the survey
- how anonymity and confidentiality will be protected
- any risks and benefits of participation
- a statement that participation is voluntary
- their right to refuse to answer any questions or stop the interview and participation in the survey at any time, without jeopardizing the services normally provided to them
- how the data will be used.

More information on the content of informed consent can be obtained from the CIOMS guidelines or the website of the WHO Ethics Review Committee (http://www.who.int/rpc/research_ethics/erc/en/index.html).

After provision of this information verbally, respondents can also be given written explanations about the survey. The person who is administering the informed consent has to be ready to explain any sections that the potential participant may not understand and should encourage participants to ask questions. The decision to participate (i.e. provide the consent) should be voluntary, and respondents must not be pressured by anyone to participate in the survey. With anonymous surveys, oral consent is obtained as a signature would breach anonymity. With oral consent, interviewers can sign a statement to verify that the respondent has been given the required information and has decided to participate. The consent is always administered by the interviewer in a private setting and may be witnessed by a second study interviewer, if necessary. Participants are free to answer the questions voluntarily and to terminate their participation in the study at any moment without suffering any consequences.

Consent of minors

In most countries, parents are required to consent to their children participating in surveys. The age at which children or young adults can give consent to participate varies according to the country. Parents may not want their children to participate in HIV surveys and may regard a child's or an adolescent's decision to participate as a sign of involvement in risky behaviour. Given the key importance of studying the sexual and drug behaviour of vulnerable young people, an ethical review committee may make an exception to the principle of parental consent, particularly if parental knowledge may place adolescents at risks of being harmed by parents. The importance of understanding patterns of sexual and drug-using behaviour among adolescents justifies studies involving adolescents who are able to understand the risks and benefits of participating.

4.7.4   Incentives

Incentives are a means of validating the importance of participation in surveillance activities by community members. Population members are giving up important personal time and contributing meaningfully to their community. Incentives should be appropriate for compensating or thanking participants for time away from work and other costs occurred (for example, costs of transport). Incentives for participation in surveillance studies should not be too high to unfairly influence participation, nor too low to make target group members uninterested in participating. Incentives may include money, tickets for transport, vouchers for mobile phones or food. The level of incentive should be explored during the pre-surveillance assessment and made in consultation with local institutional review board or other ethical committee and other researchers. Of note, using incentives can sometimes bias the sample towards those who have a greater need for the incentive.

4.7.5   Unlinked anonymous HIV testing

Unlinked anonymous HIV testing is usually done only for surveillance purposes. It is considered ethically acceptable to do unlinked anonymous testing (UAT) without informed consent if the following criteria are met:

- blood is routinely collected as part of client/patient care for a reason other than HIV testing
- personal identifiers are removed from the blood sample before HIV testing is performed
- voluntary HIV testing services should be available on site or close by for those who wish to know their HIV status.

In addition, WHO guidelines on ethical issues in surveillance state that "communities should be broadly notified that blood collected for one purpose may be anonymously tested for HIV. Although fully informed consent is not required for unlinked anonymous surveillance, the wishes of individuals wishing to opt out of such surveillance should be respected where possible." Following the surveillance, data obtained should be made public, be used to benefit the population they originate from and conveyed to the community in a way that is clearly understandable.

Ethical concerns over UAT have been debated since early in the HIV epidemic. On the one hand, those tested cannot be given the HIV test results and therefore may miss the opportunity to be referred to HIV prevention, treatment and care services. This is particularly pertinent for pregnant women attending ANC with regard to prevention of mother-to-child transmission (PMTCT) services. Pitted against these concerns is the need for high-quality data on the epidemic to formulate the appropriate response on a societal level. Ethical justification depends on conditions that may change over time and must be reviewed periodically to determine whether they no longer warrant testing without providing results to the individuals tested. A key consideration is whether high-quality data may be obtained by other methods or if the data collected from UAT provide meaningful information on the epidemic. One possibility for ANC sites is that HIV testing should be universal and therefore the PMTCT data provide an accurate estimate of HIV prevalence among pregnant women without conducting UAT.

4.7.6   Linked HIV testing and case reporting

In situations where the HIV test results are linked and given back to participants, there may be an ethical concern if that country requires name-based case notification to public health authorities. In some cases of research and IBBS, named-based reporting may be exempt from these regulations. In cases where the survey is not exempt, confidentiality needs to be strictly safeguarded, and no information is to be disclosed to anyone other than the relevant public health authorities. The ethical principle should be respected that research should not be conducted if there is any potential harm to the population studied.

4.7.7   Benefits to participants

Research ethics includes the principles of beneficence (that researchers maximize benefits to subjects) and non-maleficence (that researchers avoid or minimize harm). HIV surveillance also adheres to these principles with respect to the individual participants in surveillance activities and to society at large. An example of individual benefit is the return of HIV and STI test results and the provision of related care and preventive services. Other benefits to participants and society include:

- improving HIV prevention and care programmes
- building collaboration with most-at-risk populations
- raising public awareness of the burden of disease in the population
- reducing stigma and achieving social change
- feedback of results to the community and inclusion of target communities in dissemination of the results and intervention planning.

Appendix 4

Appendix 4.1

HIV and AIDS case reporting form for adults and adolescents aged ≥ 15 years

<table>
<tr><td colspan="2" align="center">INFORMATION ON THE REPORTING SITE</td></tr>
<tr><td>Name of reporting site</td><td></td></tr>
<tr><td>Name of reporting physician</td><td>Telephone no.:</td></tr>
<tr><td>Name of laboratory where tests were done</td><td></td></tr>
<tr><td colspan="2" align="center">INFORMATION ON PATIENTS</td></tr>
<tr><td>Patient details</td><td>Enter code[1]:

Date of birth:

Sex: ☐ M ☐ F

City of residence:</td></tr>
<tr><td>Country of birth</td><td></td></tr>
<tr><td>Probable route of infection</td><td>

1. Sex between men
In the past year estimated number of:
male partners _________________   female partners _________________

2. Injected non-prescribed drugs   Year last injected _________________

3. Heterosexual
Partner who is an injection drug user ☐
Partner who is haemophiliac or a transfusion recipient ☐
Partner who is HIV-infected ☐
Infected through heterosexual transmission, no further information ☐

4. Received blood or blood components transfusion or organ transplant   Year most recently received _________________

5. Nosocomial infection

6. Occupational

7. Other (specify):
</td></tr>
<tr><td>Pregnancy history</td><td>

1. Pregnant at diagnosis: yes ☐   no ☐
2. Previous live births: yes ☐   no ☐
</td></tr>
</table>

[1] National surveillance institutions should decide which coding system to use, and should send instructions on coding together with this form to the reporting sites. Codes can be constructed by using data such as date of birth, city of birth and initials of surname. Codes must not allow identification of individuals.

<table>
<tr><td>Reason for test</td><td colspan="2">1. Known positive partner</td><td>☐</td></tr>
<tr><td></td><td colspan="2">2. Risky behaviour</td><td>☐</td></tr>
<tr><td></td><td colspan="2">3. Blood donor</td><td>☐</td></tr>
<tr><td></td><td colspan="2">4. Antenatal</td><td>☐</td></tr>
<tr><td></td><td colspan="2">5. Visa screen</td><td>☐</td></tr>
<tr><td></td><td colspan="2">6. Symptoms</td><td>☐</td></tr>
<tr><td></td><td colspan="2">7. Other (specify):</td><td></td></tr>
</table>

HIV antibody tests used at diagnosis

1. HIV-1 EIA:

Positive ☐ Negative ☐ Not done ☐ ___|___| mm/yy

Done as: Screening ☐ Confirmatory ☐ ___|___| mm/yy

2. HIV-1/HIV-2 combination EIA

Positive ☐ Negative ☐ Not done ☐ ___|___| mm/yy

Done as: Screening ☐ Confirmatory ☐ ___|___| mm/yy

3. Western blot/immunoblot

Indeterminate ☐ Positive ☐ Negative ☐ Not done ☐ ___|___| mm/yy

4. Rapid tests (name):

Screening ☐ Confirmatory ☐ ___|___| mm/yy

Screening ☐ Confirmatory ☐ ___|___| mm/yy

HIV detection tests

1. HIV culture Positive ☐ Negative ☐ Not done ☐ ___|___| mm/yy

2. HIV antigen test Positive ☐ Negative ☐ Not done ☐ ___|___| mm/yy

3. HIV DNA PCR Positive ☐ Negative ☐ Not done ☐ ___|___| mm/yy

4. HIV RNA PCR Positive ☐ Negative ☐ Not done ☐ ___|___| mm/yy

5. Other (specify): ____

Other laboratory tests

1. CD4 count __________ (cells/mm^3) ___|___| mm/yy __________ Not done

2. CD4 percent ________ % ___|___| mm/yy __________ Not done

3. Viral load __________ (copies/ml) ___|___| mm/yy __________ Not done

WHO clinical staging of HIV infection

WHO clinical stage 1: asymptomatic ☐

WHO clinical stage 2: mild symptoms ☐

WHO clinical stage 3: advanced symptoms ☐

WHO clinical stage 4: severe symptoms ☐

Date form completed: __________|__________|__________| dd/mm/yy

Send the completed form to: ____

To be filled at the surveillance institution:

Date the form is received by the surveillance institution: __________|__________|__________| dd/mm/yy

Appendix 4.2

HIV and AIDS case reporting form for children aged <15 years

<table>
<tr><td colspan="2" align="center">INFORMATION ON THE REPORTING SITE</td></tr>
<tr><td>Name of reporting hospital or other centre or institution</td><td></td></tr>
<tr><td>Name of reporting physician</td><td>Telephone no.:</td></tr>
<tr><td>Name of laboratory where tests were done</td><td></td></tr>
<tr><td colspan="2" align="center">INFORMATION ON PATIENTS</td></tr>
<tr><td>Patient details</td><td>Enter code[1]:

Date of birth:
Sex: ☐ M ☐ F
City of residence:</td></tr>
<tr><td>Country of birth</td><td></td></tr>
<tr><td>Child's biological mother's HIV infection status</td><td>1. Diagnosed with HIV infection ☐
2. HIV status unknown ☐
3. Known to be uninfected after this child's birth ☐
4. Refused HIV testing ☐</td></tr>
<tr><td>If mother is HIV-infected, did she receive zidovudine during pregnancy?</td><td>Yes ☐ No ☐ Unknown ☐ Refused ☐
Please specify if mother received any other antiretroviral medication during pregnancy __________
____
________________________________</td></tr>
<tr><td>Before the diagnosis of HIV infection/ AIDS, this child had (tick all possible exposures)</td><td>1. Received blood or blood components transfusion or organ transplant   Year most recently received __________
2. Sexual contact with a male ☐
3. Sexual contact with a female ☐
4. Injected non-prescribed drugs ☐
5. Other (specify):</td></tr>
</table>

---

[1] National surveillance institutions should decide which coding system to use, and should send instructions on coding to reporting physicians together with this form. Codes can be constructed by using data such as date of birth, city of birth and initials of surname, or in some other way. Codes must not allow identification of individuals.

<table>
<tr><td>HIV antibody tests used at diagnosis</td><td>

1. HIV-1 EIA

Positive ☐ Negative ☐ Not done ☐ ____|____| mm/yy

Done as: Screening ☐ Confirmatory ☐ ____|____| mm/yy

2. HIV-1/ HIV-2 combination EIA

Positive ☐ Negative ☐ Not done ☐ ____|____| mm/yy

Done as: Screening ☐ Confirmatory ☐ ____|____| mm/yy

3. Western blot/immunoblot

Indeterminate ☐ Positive ☐ Negative ☐ Not done ☐ ____|____| mm/yy

4. Rapid tests (name)

Screening ☐ Confirmatory ☐ ____|____| mm/yy

Screening ☐ Confirmatory ☐ ____|____| mm/yy

</td></tr>
<tr><td>HIV detection tests</td><td>

1. HIV culture Positive ☐ Negative ☐ Not done ☐ ____|____| mm/yy

2. HIV antigen test Positive ☐ Negative ☐ Not done ☐ ____|____| mm/yy

3. HIV DNA PCR Positive ☐ Negative ☐ Not done ☐ ____|____| mm/yy

4. HIV RNA PCR Positive ☐ Negative ☐ Not done ☐ ____|____| mm/yy

5. Other (specify):

</td></tr>
<tr><td>Other laboratory tests</td><td>

1. CD4 count __________ (cells/mm^3) ____|____| mm/yy __________ Not done

2. CD4 percent ________ % ____|____| mm/yy __________ Not done

3. Viral load __________ (copies/ml) ____|____| mm/yy __________ Not done

</td></tr>
<tr><td>Clinical staging of HIV infection</td><td>

WHO clinical stage 1: asymptomatic ☐

WHO clinical stage 2: mild symptoms ☐

WHO clinical stage 3: advanced symptoms ☐

WHO clinical stage 4: severe symptoms ☐

</td></tr>
<tr><td>Date form completed:</td><td>

__________|__________|__________| dd/mm/yy

</td></tr>
</table>

Send the completed form to: ____

To be filled at the surveillance institution:

Date the form is received by the surveillance institution: __________|__________|__________| dd/mm/yy

References

1   Lee LM, Rutherford GW. Analysis and interpretation of case-based HIV surveillance data. In M'inkatha N, Lynfield R, Beneden C, de Valk H, eds. *Infectious disease surveillance*. London, Blackwell Publishers, 2007.

2   *WHO case definitions of HIV for surveillance and revised clinical staging and immunological classification of HIV-related disease in adults and children*. Geneva, WHO, 2006.

3   *Guidelines for appropriate evaluations of HIV testing technologies in Africa. Based on a workgroup meeting in Harare*. Atlanta, Georgia, WHO Regional Office for Africa/ Centers for Disease Control, 2001.

4   Kandathil AJ, Ramalingam S, Kannangai R, David S, Sridharan G. Molecular epidemiology of HIV. *Indian journal of medical research*, 2005, 121:333–44.

5   Branson BM. Rapid tests for HIV antibody. *AIDS reviews*, 2000, 2:76–83.

6   *HIV assays: operational characteristics (phase 1). Report 14. Simple/rapid tests*. Geneva, WHO, 2004.

7   *Sources and prices of selected medicines and diagnostics for people living with HIV/AIDS*, 6th ed. Cairo, UNICEF/UNAIDS/WHO/MSF, 2005.

8   McDougal JS, Pilcher CD, Parekh BS, Gershy-Damet G, Branson BM, Marsh K, Wiktor SZ. Surveillance for HIV-1 incidence using tests for recent infection in resource-constrained countries. *AIDS*, 2005, 19(suppl 2):S25–30. Review.

9   McFarland W, Busch MP, Kellogg TA, Rawal BD, Satten GA, Katz MH, Dilley J, Janssen RS. Detection of early HIV infection and estimation of incidence using a sensitive/less-sensitive enzyme immunoassay testing strategy at anonymous counseling and testing sites in San Francisco. *Journal of acquired immune deficiency syndromes*, 1999, 22(5):484–9.

10 Janssen RS, Satten GA, Stramer SL, Rawal BD, O'Brien TR, Weiblen BJ, Hecht FM, Jack N, Cleghorn FR, Kahn JO, Chessney MA, Busch MP. New testing strategy to detect early HIV-1 infection for use in incidence estimates and for clinical and prevention purposes. *Journal of the American Medical Association*, 1998, 280(1):42–8.

11 *UNAIDS reference group on estimates, modelling and projections' statement on the use of the BED-assay for the estimation of HIV-1 incidence for surveillance or epidemic monitoring*. Geneva, UNAIDS reference group on estimates, modelling and projections, 2005. Available at http://www.epidem.org/Publications/BED%20 statement.pdf.

12 *Interim recommendations for the use of the BED capture enzyme immunoassay for incidence, estimation, and surveillance.* Atlanta, Georgia, Centers for Disease Control, 2006. Available at http://www.cdc.gov/nchstp/od/GAP/pa_surveillance.htm. Accessed on 4 April 2007.

13 Karita E, Price M, Hunter E, Chomba E, Allen S, Fei L, Kamali A, Sanders EJ. Anzala O, Katende M, Ketter N, the IAVI Collaborative Seroprevalence and Incidence Study Team. Investigating the utility of the HIV-1 BED capture enzyme immunoassay using cross-sectional and longitudinal seroconverter specimens from Africa. *AIDS*, 2007, 21(4):403–8.

14 *Interpretation of the hepatitis B panel.* Atlanta, Georgia, Centers for Disease Control. Available at http://www.cdc.gov/ncidod/diseases/hepatitis/b/Bserology.htm.

15 Guidelines for laboratory testing and results reporting of antibody to hepatitis C virus. *Morbidity and mortality weekly report*, 2003, 52:RR-3.

16 *Guidelines for measuring national HIV prevalence in population-based surveys.* UNAIDS/WHO Working Group on Global HIV/AIDS and STI Surveillance. Geneva, UNAIDS/WHO, 2005.

17 *Guidelines for second generation HIV surveillance.* Geneva, WHO/UNAIDS, 2002.

18 Copas AJ, Wellings K, Erens B, Mercer CH, McManus S, Fenton KA, Korovessis C, Macdowall W, Nanchahal K, Johnson AM. The accuracy of reported sensitive sexual behaviour in Britain: exploring the extent of change 1990–2000. *Sexually transmitted infections*, 2002, 78(1):26–30.

19 Kissinger P, Rice J, Farley T, Trim S, Jewitt K, Margavio V, Martin DH. Application of computer-assisted interviews to sexual behavior research. *American journal of epidemiology*, 1999, 149(10):950–4.

Part 5

Data management, analysis and interpretation

5.1

Introduction

The overarching purpose of surveillance is to use the collected data. Formulating evidence-based policies is one example of the use of surveillance data. Repeated cross-sectional surveillance surveys and sentinel surveillance should be used to evaluate the effects and impact of HIV programmes. Together with data from surveillance surveys, operational research and case reporting help identify data gaps and ways to refine the surveillance system; for example, whether the scope of surveillance should be widened to include other groups at risk or to scale back surveillance activities that are no longer useful. Using bio-behavioural data, public health officials plan in which areas and for what priority groups it is necessary to provide prevention interventions and set goals for coverage to be achieved. Data on HIV testing uptake and barriers, also obtained from bio-behavioural surveys, can direct the scale-up of national testing programmes. Data on HIV prevalence, opportunistic infections and other measures of the burden of disease help plan for meeting current and future health care needs.

All these uses require the highest possible quality of data. This part outlines surveillance activities that occur after the data collection phase—the management, analysis and interpretation of data for programme planning.

5.2

Data management

Data management includes a range of activities to ensure the quality of data, from the recording of information on questionnaires to entry into an electronic database, the preparation of the dataset for analysis and the archiving of data for future use. Databases can be constructed, and data entry can be done using data management software packages (e.g. Microsoft Excel, Epi Info, Microsoft Access) and then transferred to a statistical analysis software package (e.g. Stata, SAS, Epi Info, R, SPSS).

Data management procedures should be detailed prior to data collection. A surveillance survey planning phase develops guidelines for all data management steps including the handling and storage of questionnaires, standardized coding of variables, data entry and database structure and storage. Data entry specialists are responsible for writing the data entry programs and data cleaning. Data management is done during several stages of the survey, including:

- data collection
- data entry
- data cleaning.

Several issues are important for data management to be effective.

- Proper data collection and storage are essential for effective data management in the field.
- Data transfer procedures and time-lines for sending data should be defined in the survey protocol, before the study is begun. Questionnaires and clinical data forms can be transported from the field according to the agreed time intervals (e.g. every day, every week or every two weeks). Laboratory data forms can be collected on a periodic basis and brought to a centralized location for data entry. In clinic-based surveillance, data collection forms are usually sent to the surveillance office/institution at the regional or national level, and data are then transferred from the forms into the database.
- The data entry template should closely follow the questionnaire structure and should be user-friendly.
- To minimize errors in entering data from paper forms to the electronic database, data are ideally entered twice by two different persons and any discrepancies are reconciled against the original paper forms. If resources are limited, a random 10% part of the data is re-entered and checked against the original data. Those who enter data should be trained in data entry and questionnaire structure.

- Before designing the database, the variables on the questionnaire need to be coded to ensure the responses are recorded in a standard manner. To this end, a well documented dictionary or code book is created to define the values of each question.
- Questionnaires and paper printouts of datasets should be stored in a locked cabinet, and electronic copies should be backed up electronically with secure password protection.

In the field, data management includes:

- training of staff on all aspects of collection of data
- timely and accurately filling out of all data collection forms (these may include forms other than the main part of the questionnaire)
- quality control (i.e. double-checking) of questionnaires for completeness and consistency of data; for example, this can be done at the end of each day by another interviewer or a supervisor, and at the end of the week by field supervisors.

In the office, responses from questionnaires should be coded, and then data should be entered into a database. Data entry templates which are used to enter and store data electronically should follow the questionnaire structure and be constructed in the way that enables automated quality control measures, such as:

- range checks (e.g. setting logical or required ranges for variables such as age between 18 and 44 years)
- logical and consistency checks (e.g. persons reporting no sex partners later reporting condom use with sex partners).

Coding of the questionnaire should be done in a consistent way and by using a standardized coding system. A data dictionary (code book) describes exactly how each variable is coded; for example: variable1_sex: 1 = male, 2 = female, 3 = unknown, 9 = unstated; variable2_age: range 18–103 years, 999-unknown). Data entry programs can also be constructed to recognize repeating codes such as:

- yes = 1, no = 0
- don't know = 999
- refused = 888
- missing = 777.

Rules also need to be established for entering answers to open-ended questions, such as entering the first 100 characters, or having supervisors classify a set of common responses.

The process of data checking and cleaning is necessary to prepare the data for analysis and is done by doing basic descriptive statistics, such as:

- range checks to assure that values are within a valid range
- review of the amount of missing data and distribution of missing data (by site, by variable, by interviewer)
- checking for duplicate records and deleting any that are found
- checking that responses are internally consistent: for example, that those who reported condom use in past 12 months also reported having sex partners during that time
- identification of responses that fall well outside of the distribution for the dataset (outliers) and assessment of their plausibility.

In a self-completed questionnaire, there may be a number of cases with many answers missing, and an assessment will need to be made regarding whether or not to include these cases in the analysis. Outliers are values that are far away from the rest of the data. It is advisable to run analysis with and without outliers to assess their impact on interpretation. The treatment of outliers (i.e. to include or collapse into categories) should be decided in consultation with the investigators and a statistician.

Finding many inconsistencies indicates a need to contact field staff to clarify issues and to check the data against the original questionnaires (which should always be retained after data entry is finished for a specified period of time). An apparent inconsistency, for example, would be if someone said that he did not use drugs in the past month, but in another question reported sharing needles during that time. In case errors are found, there is a need to go back to the questionnaire and check whether the error was made in the data entry stage or a question was not accurately answered. If there are too many answers that do not make sense for a particular individual, or a great deal of missing data, consideration should be given to discarding the data from that participant. Patterns of mistakes across participants signals lack of clarity in the questions and/or the need for further interviewer training. Finding such errors early allows for improvement of the questionnaire and data quality.

HIV test data are entered in the laboratory or at the surveillance office, and that file is merged with the file that contains data from the questionnaire so that the biological and behavioural data can be linked for the analysis. The participant's name (if such information is collected) and identification of a small enumeration area (name of a small village or another very small geographic area) should not be entered into the database that contains HIV results to preserve confidentiality. Biological and behavioural data are linked through the use of non-identifying study codes.

When data cleaning is completed, multiple copies of the dataset and a code book should be made and stored in different secure locations. For surveillance, it is particularly important to store the database and a code book for future use in the analysis of trends over several years.

5.3

Data analysis

The primary analysis of surveillance data is the examination of key measures by person, place and time. This chapter provides an overview of the main types of surveillance data analysis.

As statistical analysis is often complex, it is recommended that the reader consult a statistician and refer to a statistical textbook for further details. Knowledge of a statistical software package is also a prerequisite for analysis. Some of the more commonly used statistical programs for surveillance data analysis are Epi Info (available free at www.cdc.gov/epiinfo), Stata (www.stata.com), SPSS (www.spss.com), SAS (www.sas.com) and, for RDS data only, RDSAT (available free at www.respondentdrivensampling.org). Epi Info can perform simple analyses, while Stata, SPSS, R and SAS enable more complex analyses, including analysis of complex survey data (e.g. accounting for cluster designs and sampling weights). Data can be transferred from the management programs in which data were entered to programs for data analysis. Analysis of data often entails recoding and creation of new variables; it is therefore important that the original data file never be overwritten. Rather, a copy of the original dataset is used for analysis.

Before outlining the basic principles of surveillance data analysis, it is important to emphasize certain limitations of surveillance data. Surveillance data are descriptive in nature and are, in the majority of cases, not used for single hypothesis testing but are used to explore multiple issues affecting HIV prevalence and risk behaviour. Surveillance data are also used to generate hypotheses that can be used to guide and focus further research. Some surveillance databases contain only aggregated data; that is, cases are reported in categories for each variable separately, and it is not possible to link up all the variables pertaining to any one case, making individual-level analysis impossible. Data collected for individual case-based surveillance and community-based surveys allow individual-level analysis.

A plan for surveillance data analysis is prepared during the design stage of each survey and included in the protocol.

The first phase of data analysis includes univariate descriptive analysis, such as simple frequencies of HIV prevalence and risk behaviour overall and the calculation of means, medians and confidence intervals. As surveillance data focus on measures by person, place and time, frequencies, means and medians are also stratified by other variables of interest, such as by age group, sex or geographic area. This stratification is a form of bivariate analysis (i.e. examining two variables at a time). Analysis by person and place permits identification of disparities in disease or risk behaviour across different groups of people or regions. Analysis of place also assesses any clustering of cases by geographical area. Analysis by time assesses whether the epidemic is increasing, decreasing, or remaining stable in the long or short term (usually a minimum of three points in time are needed to assess a temporal trend).

There are two basic types of variable[1] in statistical analysis: continuous and categorical. Continuous variables are those that can take any value between a given range, such as age in years or number of sex partners, and have a clear ordered hierarchy. Categorical variables are those that can take only a limited number of responses, such as sex or level of education completed. A ranking or order may (ordinal) or may not (nominal) be present. Ordinal variables have a natural hierarchy (i.e. level of education) while nominal variables do not have an inherent hierarchy (i.e. sex).

Example of continuous variables

- Number of sex partners, age, CD4+ cell count, number of times injecting equipment was shared in the past month.

Example of categorical variables

- Nominal: HIV status, sex, ethnicity, occupation, language, condom use at most recent intercourse.
- Ordinal: educational level, HIV knowledge score.

As evident above, continuous variables can be made into ordinal categorical variables. For example, we often recode continuous age into categories for stratified analysis using groups such as 15–19 years, 20–24, 25–29, etc. HIV prevalence is then expressed according to age group, with prevalence among younger people used as a proxy for more recent HIV infection or incidence.

For analysis, variables are also classified as exposure (independent) and outcome (dependent) variables, for example when looking at relationships between certain behaviour (number of partners, condom use) and diseases (HIV prevalence, STI prevalence).

Examples of exposure (predictor or independent) variables

- Age group, sex, number of partners in the past year, always using condoms in commercial sex activities in the past week.

Examples of outcome (dependent) variables

- HIV prevalence, STI prevalence, always using condoms in commercial sex activities during the past week (note here that it can also be a behavioural outcome of interest).

There are three main types of analysis that are done with each wave of a surveillance survey: univariate, bivariate and multivariate. An outline of these types of analysis is provided in the following sections.

---

[1]   A variable is a characteristic that can be measured, such as proportion of population living with HIV, or condom use with paying partners.

Adjustment for non-response is another key issue in the analysis of the survey data, and a method of adjustment of the HIV prevalence for non-response is described in chapter 5.4.

5.3.1 Univariate analysis

Most of indicators defined for surveillance purposes are calculated through univariate analysis, which is the examination of the distribution of one variable only. Such variables can be, for example, the proportion of participants who are HIV-infected or the proportion of injection drug users who shared injecting equipment at least once during the past month. Univariate analysis constructs the point estimates (e.g. proportion, mean) for indicators along with associated 95% confidence intervals (CI) based on the standard error (SE). The SE of a proportion, for example, is calculated as follows:

$$\mathrm{SE} = \sqrt{\frac{p\,(100-p)}{n}}$$

where p = proportion (expressed as %); n = the sample size in the denominator of the indicator.

$$95\%\ \mathrm{CI} = p \pm (\mathrm{SE} \times 1.96)$$

The larger the sample size, the narrower and more precise the confidence intervals are. However, larger samples are more costly, hence one has to decide how narrow a confidence interval is justifiable.

The following measures can be described in univariate analysis:

- number of observations, proportion of missing values
- point prevalence and 95% CI for categorical variables, e.g. HIV, STI and behavioural measures
- mean, standard deviation and 95% CI for continuous variables, e.g. age in years ± years
- median, range of values, interquartile range, e.g. median number of partners, 25th percentile, 75th percentile.

5.3.2 Bivariate analysis

Bivariate analysis examines two variables at a time (e.g. HIV prevalence by sex).

Bivariate analysis is often presented in 2 × 2 tables, when both variables have only two categories (Table 5.1) and can be used to test for the association between an exposure or predictor and an outcome. A test commonly used to measure the association between two categorical variables is the chi-square test. The chi-square test compares the observed numbers in each of the four categories in the table (Table 5.1) with the expected numbers, assuming that there was no difference in the number of partners according to whether someone had same sex partners. By calculating the p-value, we can estimate the probability that the observed association was due to chance. The usual cut-off point is taken as 0.05 which means that if the p-value is less than 0.05, there is less than 5% probability that the observed association occurred by chance (and so we assume there is a genuine association between the two variables). The tables and formulas used in chi-square statistics can be found in most books on statistics.

Table 5.1 shows an example of bivariate analysis from a household-based survey on sexual health among young people in Croatia [1]. The outcome variable in this example is "total number of partners in life", split into two categories, and the exposure variable is stratified in two categories as "had only heterosexual partners" or "also had partners of the same sex". The results show that young men who had partners of the same sex reported significantly more frequently more than five partners in life (59.9%) compared to those who had only heterosexual partners (20.6%). A *p*-value of < 0.001 means that there is less than 0.1% chance that there is no effect of the exposure variable (having partners of the same sex) on the outcome (having more than five partners in life). Because of this small probability, we interpret the results of the bivariate analysis to mean that there is a significant association between having partners of the same sex and the reporting of more than five partners in life. The *p*-value of less than 0.05 is an arbitrary convention that denotes there is a statistically significant association (at the 5% probability level). It is useful to always show the actual *p*-value, and not just whether it is larger or smaller than 0.05.

Another statistical test for comparing two proportions is the *Z*-statistic. For example, the test can determine if the difference between two proportions from two surveillance sites is statistically significant (Table 5.2). Before calculating whether there are significant differences in prevalence between two sites, it is best to directly standardize (weight) the data based on the standard population age distribution from the census data. Direct

Table 5.1 Example of bivariate data analysis: reporting of an STI-related symptom among men aged 18–24

	Total number of partners in life: 1–4	**More than 5 partners in life**	**Total**
Had only heterosexual partners	301 (79.4%)	78 (20.6%)	379 (100%)
Had partners of same sex	12 (40.1%)	17 (59.9%)	29 (100%)
Total	313 (76.6%)	95 (23.4%)	408 (100%)

Source: Štulhofer A, Ajduković D, Božičević I, Kufrin K. *HIV/AIDS and youth in Croatia. The study of sexual behaviour, practices and attitudes. Final report* [in Croatian]. Zagreb, Ministry of Health, 2006.
Chi-square = 22.05; *p* < 0.001

Table 5.2 Example of calculation of Z-statistic for two proportions

Sample	**Number of persons tested**	**Number of persons HIV-positive**	**Estimated HIV prevalence**
1	n_1	x_1	$P_1 = x_1/n_1$
2	n_2	x_2	$P_2 = x_2/n_2$
Combined	$n\ (= n_1 + n_2)$	$x\ (= x_1 + x_2)$	$P = x/n$

standardization takes into account different age structures of two sentinel sites. For further information on direct standardization and other tests mentioned here, see statistical textbooks such as Hennekens CH, Buring JE. *Epidemiology in medicine.* Boston, Little, Brown and Company, 1987.

Tables in statistical textbooks provide the *p*-values associated with different values for the *Z*-statistic. The formula for calculating the *Z*-statistic is:

$$Z = \frac{\left| P_2 - P_1 \right| - \dfrac{1}{2}\left(\dfrac{1}{n_1} + \dfrac{1}{n_2}\right)}{\sqrt{P(1-P) \times \left(\dfrac{1}{n_1} + \dfrac{1}{n_2}\right)}}$$

If the *p*-value is less than 0.05, one may conclude that there is a significant difference in the HIV prevalence for the populations represented by the two samples.

For assessing the relationship between a categorical predictor variable and a continuous outcome variable, the *t*-test can be used. If both a predictor and an outcome are continuous variables, linear regression can be used. While details of conducting *t*-tests and linear regression are beyond the scope of this manual, details on these procedures can be found in all biostatistics and epidemiology texts (for example, Jewell NP. *Statistics for epidemiology.* Boca Raton, Florida, Chapman & Hall, 2004.)

Analysis of temporal trends

Repeated surveillance survey waves permit the assessment of changes in the epidemic over time. A change is possible to assess between two survey waves; however, ideally three waves are the minimum needed to determine a temporal trend. The main aim of trend analysis is to assess whether HIV prevalence (or other outcome of interest) has been increasing or decreasing or remains stable over time. If there are interventions being implemented in these population groups, the trend analysis can help assess whether these interventions are having any impact (however, the analysis does not prove that the interventions are necessarily the cause of the trend). Trends in HIV prevalence can be analysed if the surveillance surveys have been carried out using the same methods, at the same sites and on the same population groups over time. It is advisable to assess trends separately by site; aggregating data from different sites should only be done if sociodemographic characteristics and population catchment areas are similar or with statistical adjustments or standardization (an example is provided below).

Analysis of trend commonly uses the chi-square test for linear trend. The most effective way to present temporal trend data is graphically (site by site), year by year. Epi Info EpiTable functions can calculate the chi-square test for linear trend[1].

The results indicate the value of chi-square for slope, and the respective *p*-value, which can be compared with the value of *p* = 0.05. If the *p*-value is less than 0.05, it can be concluded that the prevalence is changing significantly over time (either decreasing or increasing). The chi-square test for linear trend is based on the assumption that the

---

[1]   *Guidelines for conducting HIV sentinel serosurveys among pregnant women and other groups.* Geneva, UNAIDS/ WHO, 2003.

change in prevalence is linear. This assumption of linearity should be checked by carrying out the chi-square test of linearity and by visual inspection of the graphed line (i.e. do the points fall on a line that rises or falls steadily?). A p-value of this test of less 0.05 does not necessarily mean the assumption of linearity is valid.

The calculation of 95% CI also provides an estimate of whether or not the change in behaviour or HIV prevalence in two survey rounds is significant by examining if they overlap each other. For example, we can take a hypothetical survey in which in 2002, 35% of lorry drivers reported using condoms with sex workers during the past year, and in 2005 that proportion increased to 45% We have calculated 95% CI to be: 31%–39% in 2002 and 41%–49% in 2005. Since the confidence intervals do not overlap, we can say that the change was not due to random error, i.e. that a significantly higher proportion of lorry drivers used condoms in 2005. This conclusion is valid only if both surveys done in 2002 and 2005 used the same sampling method and were probability-based samples.

5.3.3   Multivariate analysis

Multivariate analysis examines two or more variables simultaneously. For much surveillance data, multivariate analysis is done by regression modelling, which enables the estimation of the effect of selected explanatory variables on the outcomes adjusted for the effects of other explanatory variables. This adjustment separates the effects of each predictor variable (e.g. HIV-prevalence can be related to both condom use and number of partners) as well as adjusting for confounders or variables that mask or apparently enhance effects (e.g. age may be a confounder in the relationship between HIV infection and marital status). Multivariate analysis is done with statistical software packages such as SPSS, Stata and SAS.

When the outcome is dichotomous (e.g. HIV-positive or negative) then the type of regression analysis can be logistic regression. The outcomes of logistic regression analysis are expressed as **odds ratios**, which compare one or more categories of an exposure variable to the baseline (the baseline group has an odds ratio equal to 1.0), according to the main outcome of interest. Odds ratios are measures of the strength of association.

As an example, the type of question that can be answered with multivariate logistic regression analysis is "are those who have been imprisoned for more than six months more or less likely to be HIV-positive, after adjusting for drug use before imprisonment?" If we get an odds ratio (OR) of 1.4, this means that those imprisoned longer than six months have a 40% higher chance than those imprisoned for less than six months of being HIV-positive, after adjusting for drug behaviour before imprisonment (the odds ratio should then be referred to as an adjusted odds ratio, i.e. AOR). 95% CI and p-values are calculated for each OR.

The odds ratio is calculated as shown in the table below: the odds of outcome in the exposed group ÷ odds of outcome in the unexposed group.

Odds of outcome among the exposed = number with outcome among the exposed (a) ÷ number who did not develop outcome among the exposed (b).

Odds of outcome among the unexposed = number with outcome among the unexposed (c) ÷ number who did not develop outcome among the unexposed (d).

Predictor variable (exposure)	Outcome variable		Total
	Present	**Absent**	
Present	a	b	$a + b$
Absent	c	d	$c + d$
Total	$a + c$	$b + d$	n

$$\text{OR} = \frac{a \times d}{b \times c}$$

Odds ratio is interpreted as:

- OR = 1.0; no effect
- OR > 1.0; effect, greater odds of outcome with the predictor (i.e. risk for infection)
- OR < 1.0; effect, lower odds of outcome with the predictor (i.e. a protective effect).

Confidence intervals that include the value 1.0 indicate no effect (i.e. p-value > 0.05).

It is always important to bear in mind that a statistically significant association does not necessarily prove causation. The following factors strengthen the likelihood of causality:

- temporal association: the predictor variable precedes the outcome variable in time
- strength of association: larger odds ratios favour causality over smaller ones
- biological plausibility: there is a scientific explanation for the association
- consistency: the association observed in different studies with different designs
- dose-response: the strength of association increases as exposure to predictor increases.

5.3.4 Weighting of infection rates (direct standardization)

HIV prevalence rates are strongly related to age and sex; i.e. HIV prevalence strongly depends on the age–sex composition of the population. Analysis of data from clinic-based sentinel sites often requires standardization because of differences in sociodemographic structure between clinic attenders. It is therefore inaccurate to use overall prevalence when comparing different sites unless they have the same age–sex structure. If we want to compare prevalence rates from different sites, we need to first weight the samples, i.e. perform direct standardization of the data. In direct standardization, the age-specific rates from the populations under study are applied to a standard population, resulting in standardized rates. The standard population can be the census population from the local area or the whole country.

An example of direct standardization is provided below, adapted from the example provided in *Guidelines for conducting HIV sentinel serosurveys among pregnant women and other groups*. Geneva, UNAIDS/WHO, 2003.

HIV prevalence in ANC clinic A

Age (years)	Number tested	Number HIV-positive	Age-specific HIV prevalence (%)
15–19	75	4	5.3
20–24	101	7	6.9
25–29	50	4	8.0
30–34	62	3	4.8
35–39	53	2	3.8
40–44	45	1	2.2
45–49	74	2	2.7
Total	460	23	5.0

Crude prevalence in clinic A: 23/460 × 100 = 5.0%.

HIV prevalence in ANC clinic B

Age (years)	Number tested	Number HIV-positive	Age-specific HIV prevalence (%)
15–19	35	1	2.9
20–24	45	1	2.2
25–29	50	2	4.0
30–34	65	0	0
35–39	92	7	7.6
40–44	38	3	7.9
45–49	61	2	3.3
Total	386	16	4.1

Crude prevalence in clinic B: 16/386 × 100 = 4.1%

Census data for women in the country

Age (years)	Population
15–19	90 000
20–24	100 000
25–29	110 000
30–34	100 000
35–39	80 000
40–44	60 000
45–49	50 000
Total	590 000

Standardized prevalence rates for clinic A

Age (years)	Population number	Age-specific prevalence in clinic A (%)	Expected number of HIV infections
15–19	90 000	5.3	4 770
20–24	100 000	6.9	6 900
25–29	110 000	8.0	8 800
30–34	100 000	4.8	4 800
35–39	80 000	3.8	3 040
40–44	60 000	2.2	1 320
45–49	50 000	2.7	1 350
Total	590 000	5.3	30 980

Standardized prevalence rates for clinic B

Age (years)	Population number	Age-specific prevalence in clinic B (%)	Expected number of HIV infections
15–19	90 000	2.9	2 610
20–24	100 000	2.2	2 200
25–29	110 000	4.0	4 400
30–34	100 000	0	0
35–39	80 000	7.6	6 080
40–44	60 000	7.9	4 740
45–49	50 000	3.3	1 650
Total	590 000	3.7	21 680

The total age-weighted prevalence for clinics A and B are calculated as: the expected number of HIV infections/total population of 15–49 years olds × 100%.

The standardized HIV prevalence for clinic A is 30 980/590 000 = 5.3%, and for clinic B it is 21 680/590 000 = 3.7%. These two rates are slightly different from those calculated as site-specific rates. The advantage is that once standardized, the two rates can be directly compared with each other.

In surveys using cluster-based sampling with a design effect and where subpopulation members had unequal probabilities of selection, cluster-weighted analysis has to be performed. The clustering or design effect can alter the SE for estimates while unequal sampling probabilities can change the point estimates and SE. Software packages such as SPSS and Stata can be used to perform weighted analysis. Calculations of standard errors for complex survey designs that include stratification, cluster sampling and multiple stages of sample selection should be made by an experienced statistician, and the methods to do this are beyond the scope of these guidelines.

5.3.5 Using data for HIV projections and estimates modelling

UNAIDS, WHO and the UNAIDS Reference Group on Estimates, Modelling and Projections have developed software packages, including Spectrum and the Estimation and Projection Package (http://www.unaids.org/en/KnowledgeCentre/HIVData/Epidemiology/episoftware.asp) that enable calculations of national estimates of HIV prevalence based on several data sources.

In countries with a low-level or concentrated epidemic, national estimates of HIV prevalence are primarily based on surveillance data collected from populations at high risk (commercial sex workers, men who have sex with men, injection drug users) and estimates of the size of populations at high and low risk. This information is entered into point prevalence and projection spreadsheet models (called the workbook method) to find the best fitting curve that describes the evolution of adult HIV prevalence over time [2]. This adult prevalence curve, along with the national population estimates and epidemiological assumptions, is then entered into the Spectrum software to calculate the number of people infected, new infections and deaths caused by AIDS.

In countries or areas with a generalized epidemic, national estimates of HIV prevalence are based on data generated by surveillance systems that focus on pregnant women who attend sentinel ANC clinics. These data are entered into the Estimation and Projection Package (EPP) software, which uses a simple epidemiological model to find the best fitting curve that describes the evolution of adult HIV prevalence over time [3]. For each sub-epidemic defined by the user, the EPP fits a simple epidemic model to a full set of HIV surveillance data points collected from ANC over time. The fits to individual sub-epidemics are applied to the populations assigned by the user to produce the prevalence estimates and trends in the overall national epidemic. This adult prevalence curve, along with national population estimates and epidemiological assumptions, is then entered into Spectrum to calculate the number of people infected, new infections and deaths caused by AIDS. HIV prevalence estimates from population-based surveys can be used to calibrate the HIV prevalence levels obtained from ANC sites in EPP.

More detailed explanations of these methods can be found on the website of the UNAIDS Reference Group on Estimates, Modelling and Projections at http://www.epidem.org/Default.htm.

There are a number of challenges when calculating the number of people living with HIV and applying local data on HIV prevalence to the national level. Data collected from surveillance studies in low-level and concentrated epidemics are often not representative as they are mainly collected from the high-risk urban areas. The estimation of the size of most-at-risk populations is particularly challenging as few data exist in this area. WHO estimates that the prevalence of currently active men who have sex with men is in the range of 2%–5% (a point estimate of 3%) for the regions of Asia, Latin America and Caribbean, and Europe; however, for countries of the Middle East and North Africa such estimates are not available. The typical prevalence range for female sex workers is 0.3%–1.5%, though it can vary significantly between regions. The estimates of the number of clients of sex workers are in the range of 2%–5% of the adult male population (for Europe, Middle East and North Africa) [4].

5.3.6   Concepts in analysis of RDS data

The analysis of data obtained by respondent-driven sampling (RDS) is an area of active development, and changes in approaches and software are anticipated. For the present, we present the analysis of RDS data using the respondent-driven sampling analysis tool, RDSAT, and some understanding of the theoretical background of RDS related to analysis. Currently, the analysis of RDS data in RDSAT is limited to the calculation of proportions with associated confidence intervals and stratified analysis. There are efforts currently under way to improve the analytical capabilities of RDSAT. The software packages Respondent Driven Sampling Coupon Manager (RDSCM) and RDSAT and the related manuals that describe how to do data management and analysis can be downloaded free from www.respondentdrivensampling.org.

RDSAT estimates what the sample composition would have been if all groups were recruited equally effectively and if all groups possessed equal homophily[1] [5]. Essentially, RDS estimates the probability that a person of one type will recruit a person of another or the same type. It weights sample units by the inverse of their probability of selection, so units with a smaller chance of being selected have more weight. For example, RDSAT will estimate the probability that a person who is HIV-positive will recruit a person of another or same type (HIV-negative or HIV-positive) and combines it with the self-reported network size. These measures are combined to calculate the population proportion estimates.

Data requirements for RDS analysis

There are three types of data which are essential for analysis, and RDS analysis cannot be performed without this information for each respondent:

- network size—the number of people a respondent knows in the target population and that meet the selection criteria for the survey
- serial number of the coupon every respondent was recruited with
- a respondent's recruiting serial numbers—the serial numbers of the coupons the respondent gave to other recruits who entered the study.

RDSAT calculates the following parameters[2].

- Sample proportion estimate (SPE). Calculated by dividing the number of respondents with the outcome of interest by the total sample size. For instance, the proportion of individuals in the sample who are HIV-positive is the number of HIV-positives in the sample divided by the total sample size. SPE is not representative of the population because it is calculated without weighting.
- Population proportion estimate (PPE). These are estimates of proportions that are made using RDS theory and should be representative of the target populations. This is the most appropriate estimate for describing the outcome of interest (indicators). PPE are a correction for the difference between the composition of the sample and the composition of the target population.

---

[1]   Homophily indicates that people in the same network may be more similar to each other than they are to people in other networks. This characteristic is also found in cluster-based sampling where people within clusters may be more similar to each other than to those in other clusters.

[2]   Source: Johnston LG. *Conducting respondent driven sampling (RDS) studies in diverse settings: a training manual for planning RDS studies*. Atlanta, Georgia, Centers for Disease Control, 2007.

- Equilibrium proportion estimate (EPE). Estimate of the sample proportion at the time of equilibrium without accounting for differences in network sizes—it is usually achieved by wave four or five. Reaching equilibrium indicates that the sample is unbiased by the non-random selection of seeds. Equilibrium is the state whereby no more sample variation will occur irrespective of how many more waves are recruited. Recruitment chains must be long enough to reach equilibrium to ensure that the bias introduced from the initial selection of seeds is eliminated. The point at which equilibrium is reached is usually set to within 2% of the sample no longer changing.

SPE within 1–3 points of the EPE suggest that there is minimal bias introduced from the choice of seeds selected in the sample and that the theoretical expectations of the sample recruitment process correspond to the underlying theories that are the basis for RDS. When the SPE are similar to the PPE and when both estimates fall within the confidence intervals, there is minimal bias in the sample.

In brief:

- RDSAT uses network sizes and recruitment patterns to derive proportion estimates
- the RDSAT database must have links between recruiters and recruits
- data are weighted so that those with larger network sizes are given less weight
- RDSAT uses bootstrapping to produce proportion estimates.

For further information on how to conduct RDS data analysis see: Johnston LG. *Conducting respondent driven sampling (RDS) studies in diverse settings: a training manual for planning RDS studies.* Atlanta, Georgia, Centers for Disease Control, 2007. Available at http://lisagjohnston.com/user/image/final-version-of-rds-manual-2008.pdf and www. respondentdrivensampling.org.

5.4

Interpretation of data

HIV surveillance surveys seek to obtain results that are reliable and valid, can be generalized to target populations and can be used for planning of prevention and care programmes.

The epidemiology of HIV involves complex interactions that affect interpretation of surveillance data. Risk factors for transmission involve behavioural characteristics of an individual (rate of partner change, concurrent partnerships), population-level characteristics (prevalence of infection and density of sexual networks), availability and accessibility of health care, and quality of health services. Behavioural data help to interpret changes in HIV prevalence [6]. However, because behaviour precedes HIV infection [7], recent risk behaviour is not necessarily related to current HIV status as infection may have occurred some time ago.

The ability to interpret the epidemic at the national level depends on the comprehensiveness and the quality of the system's data sources. Each data source has its own advantages and disadvantages, and describing these in the surveillance reports will help to assess and compare the results of and the gaps in these multiple data sources and to interpret dynamics of HIV epidemics with greater accuracy.

Various skills are needed to synthesize biological and behavioural data, and this is often the task of a multidisciplinary team consisting of epidemiologists, public health experts, behavioural scientists and statisticians. As mentioned, it is difficult to make a direct link between current behaviour and current HIV prevalence due to the long period of time that someone may be infected with HIV. Data on some STI may be more closely linked to current behaviour, as bacterial STI have shorter incubation periods. Another option is to measure HIV incidence, which enables the estimation of current or recent HIV transmission patterns. However, the measurement of HIV incidence is challenging.

In interpreting HIV surveillance data for intervention planning, consider the following questions.

- What is the HIV prevalence obtained from surveillance surveys in the country? Which regions have the highest and lowest prevalence?
- What behaviour is most strongly associated with HIV infection?
- What population is currently the source of most infections? Which have the highest levels of risk behaviour?

- How is the epidemic changing over time? Is HIV prevalence rising, falling or remaining stable? In which populations or areas?
- What is the impact of the epidemic on individuals (e.g. morbidity and mortality)? On families? On society?
- Where should efforts be focused to produce maximum effect?
- Where should efforts be focused to ensure coverage with interventions?

Surveillance data should prompt discussion on the successes and failures of the national HIV response when interpreted along with other sources of information. Broad discussion should address the following questions.

- What worked? What didn't?
- What are the gaps and what data are currently missing?
- What needs to be added/strengthened?
- What needs to be discarded?
- What additional information do we need and can it be obtained by operational research? Qualitative methods? Refocusing HIV and behavioural surveys to other populations and/or geographical areas?

The use of surveillance data in the context of other sources of information is sometimes referred to as **triangulation**. Triangulation is broadly defined as synthesis and integration of data from multiple sources for programme decision-making [8]. Further details of how triangulation can be conducted is available at http://globalhealthsciences.ucsf.edu/PPHG/assets/docs/oms-HIV-triangulation-guide.pdf.

Triangulation of different data sources enables one to interpret surveillance information with greater confidence and accuracy compared to its interpretation alone. Triangulation also enables better assessment on levels and direction of bias. Triangulation can be effective when there are multiple data collection systems (including both quantitative and qualitative data from various sources such as research studies, programmes and surveillance) that cannot be directly combined into one dataset. Data triangulation can be used to answer different questions, ranging from explaining the trends and the levels of an HIV epidemic to assessing the population impact of HIV prevention and treatment programmes. Examples of datasets that can be included in triangulation include:

- community-based surveillance surveys, such as surveys using probability-based methods (demographic and health surveys, AIDS indicator surveys) or quasi probability-based (respondent-driven sampling surveys, time-location sampling)
- clinic-based sentinel surveillance, such as those carried out in ANC, TB or STI clinics
- programmatic data coming from VCT or PMTCT sites
- ART programme data
- HIV, AIDS, STI and TB case registries
- mortality data
- census data (population estimates)
- research studies, qualitative and quantitative.

Expert and stakeholder opinion can also be taken into account in triangulation.

Some examples of the questions that can be answered by data triangulation are as follows.

Tracking the epidemic

- Is the incidence of HIV among men who have sex with men going up or down or staying at the same level in the era of ART rollout? Among IDU? Among FSW?
- What contribution do in-country migrations make to the HIV epidemic?
- What is the impact of ART scale-up on HIV incidence?

Measuring the effect of interventions[1]

- What is the overall impact of ART programmes on adult mortality?
- What is the overall impact of PMTCT programmes on infant mortality?
- What is the overall impact of national prevention programmes on the HIV epidemic?

Coverage with interventions

- What is the current coverage of prevention and treatment interventions among injection drug users in a specific city or province and what are the gaps? Among MSM? Among FSW?
- What is the reach and intensity of HIV prevention programmes in a specific province over a given period?

Random error and bias

Random error and various biases need to be considered when interpreting surveillance data. For example, trends in HIV may be influenced by real changes in the epidemiology of the infection and/or changes in availability and access to testing, changes in the quality of surveillance systems (including better-quality sampling) and better HIV tests. Interpretation of data from the case reporting system, as well as other surveillance data, should be made within the context of prevention and control programmes and the characteristics of the health care system. Some of the issues that affect the way data are interpreted are health care–seeking practices, availability of health care services, reporting practices of health care staff (for example, high staff turnover will usually endanger system stability and quality of data), errors in the data and changes in case definitions.

During data interpretation, we need to assess and acknowledge any limitations and problems during data collection such as incomplete reporting and delays in reporting. Behavioural data often suffer from lower validity, as much behaviour of interest is intimate or stigmatized, and respondents might have not answered accurately. The quality of biological data will depend on specimen handling, transport and testing; and any problems encountered in this respect should be reported. It is difficult to estimate how representative samples are of hard-to-reach priority populations, and all methods may miss hidden pockets. It is also difficult to compare data over time and across different sites when there are differences in design of the surveillance activities, different levels of quality of data and different types of population covered [9]. This is why every attempt should be made to achieve consistent data collection mechanisms that include the same definitions of most-at-risk populations and the same data collection instruments over time.

---

[1] Here mortality can be taken as the primary indicator. This is not supposed to be a study that evaluates the effectiveness of interventions: if so the study design would need to be different.

Results from the surveys need to take into account non-systematic (random) and systematic error (bias). Random error is the type of error that results from chance and leads to imprecise results, and is related to the sample size. The larger the sample size, the less likely random error will occur. As mentioned earlier, when we obtain the value of one variable from the survey data, it is only the estimated value of that variable, and statistics can help us estimate how precise that estimate is (defined by the 95% confidence interval). Bias is the error in sampling and measurements that leads to incorrect estimates. Statistics can rarely reduce or correct for bias. Instead, proper study design and rigorous implementation are the best ways to reduce bias. The main types of bias are measurement bias, response bias and selection bias.

Measurement bias

Measurement bias occurs when the data collected do not accurately measure the characteristics of interest, which affects the validity of the data. In observational studies, measurement error can come from:

- errors in the questionnaire
- interviewer error
- respondent error
- errors in laboratory diagnostics.

Error in the questionnaire can be due to culturally inappropriate questions, questions that are not precise (e.g. "have you had unsafe sex in the last month?"), inappropriate ordering of questions and too many questions, which can exhaust a respondent.

Interviewer errors occur when an interviewer is not following the protocol, skips questions, inaccurately records the answers or does not understand a respondent (for example, if a respondent uses slang).

Respondent errors can be due to not understanding questions or deliberately giving inaccurate answers.

Laboratory errors can be due to:

- problems during specimen storage and transport which reduce the quality of a specimen
- poor laboratory technique
- using tests whose expiry date has passed or which are not valid for other reasons.

Additional laboratory issues that are relevant for data interpretation are as follows.

Using tests with improved sensitivity (e.g. switching from EIA to PCR in diagnosis of chlamydia) will yield more positives simply because more are detected. This increase does not mean that there has been an increase in the number of infections, but rather an increase in the number of **diagnosed** infections.

Using tests with better specificity might lead to higher positive predictive value (i.e. lower numbers of false positives) and therefore lower HIV prevalence in subsequent surveillance rounds. Again, the change is due to using better quality tests and not to real changes in HIV prevalence

Measurement bias can be reduced by:

- using standardized and field-tested questionnaires
- pre-testing of a questionnaire and adapting as necessary
- training and supervision of staff
- timely editing and coding of questionnaires
- using quality control measures during data collection, processing and analysis.

Response bias

In all surveys for HIV, bias due to non-response is an important issue created by differences among people's willingness and ability to be in the study.

Non-responders are always of interest for data interpretation since they may have different characteristics from responders (for example, they might be at greater or lower risk of HIV infection). Therefore, it is important to collect data on the characteristics of non-responders and to record the extent and reasons for non-participation, along with basic sociodemographic information. Non-response may be related to movement out of the place of residence or any kind of temporary absence. Non-response may be also due to refusing to participate, which can be because people already know their HIV status, for example, or they fear that they might be HIV-infected. In these cases, HIV prevalence estimates of the survey may be biased downwards by their non-response.

Assessment of, and when possible adjustment for, non-response bias is essential to interpreting survey data. One adjustment is the use of information on the characteristics of non-respondents (if available) that is used with the HIV prevalence among those who were tested to produce expected numbers of infected among those who were not tested. New estimates of prevalence are obtained by adding the expected number of infections among non-respondents to the known infections among those who were tested. In countries that carried out national population-based surveys for HIV and where the non-response was significant, the adjusted prevalence was often very different from the observed [10]. The adjustment for non-response by standardization based on age distribution, province and residence is described in *Guidelines for measuring national HIV prevalence in population-based surveys.* Geneva, UNAIDS/WHO, 2005. Available at http:// www.who.int/HIV/pub/surveillance/guidelinesmeasuringpopulation.pdf.

Selection bias

Selection biases arise when the site or area used to sample persons is not representative of the whole population of interest, for example:

- those who visit clinics included in sentinel surveillance might not be representative of the broader population
- selecting the most visible persons to participate in a surveillance survey, such as male sex workers in an MSM survey.

As mentioned previously, HIV prevalence in young pregnant women at ANC sites may overestimate HIV prevalence among women in the same age group in the general population as not all young women are sexually active. On the other hand, HIV prevalence among older pregnant women may underestimate that of other women in the same age group in the general population due to lower fertility among HIV-infected older women. HIV prevalence in rural areas measured in population-based surveys may be different from rural prevalence measured in ANC surveys because more remote and less densely populated areas are often not covered by ANC. Comparison of data from countries with generalized epidemics found on average that HIV prevalence in population-based surveys was 20% lower than in ANC sentinel surveillance [5].

Confounders

A confounder is a variable that is independently associated with both the exposure and the outcome and can falsely lead to the interpretation that the exposure is association with the outcome. Confounders can be controlled for in stratified and multivariate analysis. Common confounders are sex, age and socioeconomic status. For example, age might be associated with HIV infection, and older age may also be associated with a lower number of annual sex partners. Therefore, age confounds the relationship between the annual number of sex partners and HIV infection.

Although changes in HIV prevalence may reflect the long-term impact of multiple interventions, it is very difficult to prove that decreasing prevalence resulted from specific interventions. Other factors such as mortality, migration or the saturation of the epidemic may also explain such changes. Surveillance cannot tell us that any specific interventions have caused changes in behaviour or HIV prevalence. Targeted evaluation studies with appropriate methods (for example, community-based randomized controlled trials) should be designed for conducting evaluations of specific interventions. As mentioned earlier, triangulation of data from different sources and bringing together biological and behavioural data help to explain the trends in the epidemic and the contribution of different risk groups to the observed changes and the epidemic's likely future course. Surveillance provides us with a basis to assess past failures and successes and, vitally, to suggest any need for redirecting prevention efforts in a way that reflects the dynamics of HIV transmission.

5.5

Using surveillance data to plan appropriate HIV prevention and control programmes

HIV surveillance data are used to guide the national and local responses to the epidemic, inform programme planning (i.e. what interventions are needed, when and where) and monitor the global impact that the interventions have on the HIV epidemic. In particular, understanding the sources of new infections enables programmes to refocus efforts on geographical areas and groups at highest risk [11]. The guidelines of the Council for International Organizations of Medical Sciences emphasize that there is an ethical responsibility to use data by stating "it is not sufficient simply to determine that a disease is prevalent in the population and that new or further research is needed. The ethical requirement of 'responsiveness' can be fulfilled only if successful interventions or other kinds of benefits are made available to the population" [12].

Here we provide an example from Pakistan on how surveillance data can be used to plan programmatic responses and assess their effectiveness[1].

Example: community-based bio-behavioural surveillance surveys in Karachi and Lahore, Pakistan

In collaboration with the National AIDS Control Programme in Pakistan, Family Health International carried out cross-sectional bio-behavioural surveys in 2005 in Karachi and Lahore[2]. Surveys were carried out in groups identified to be at the highest risk of infection, and these were injection drug users, male and female sex workers, *hijra* and lorry drivers.

Data obtained from these surveys in 2005 indicate that a higher proportion of injection drug users were in contact with services providing interventions (24% in Karachi and 62% in Lahore) compared to other groups (only 3% of female sex workers in Karachi and 8% in Lahore, with even lower proportions in other risk groups). Only 10% of injection

---

[1] The example is taken from the report: *National study of reproductive tract and sexually transmitted infections.* Islamabad, National AIDS Control Programme, Ministry of Health, Government of Pakistan, 2005.
[2] The interventions asked for were: education about HIV, condom distribution, STI treatment and needle exchange.

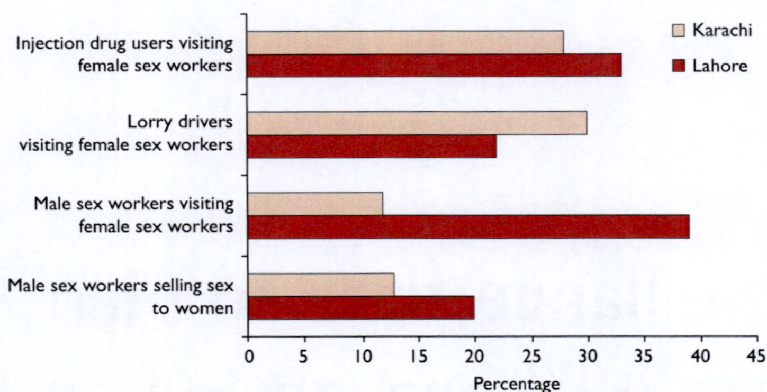

Figure 5.1 Commercial male–female sexual contacts in the past month

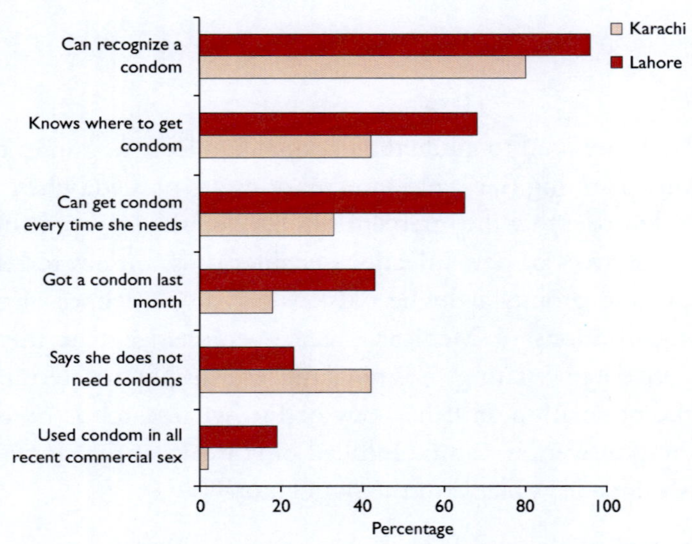

Figure 5.2 Knowledge of, access to and use of condoms among female sex workers, Pakistan

drug users had ever been tested for HIV, which indicates a very low testing uptake. HIV prevalence in this group was 23% in Karachi, which indicates a need to increase the number of VCT and needle exchange services. It was also found that, on average, drug users were injecting 65 times per month, which can be used to estimate the total number of needles that harm reduction programmes need to deliver in Karachi and Lahore when combined with estimates of the size of population of injection drug users.

Behavioural data collected in the same survey are very informative regarding the extent to which different risk groups are interlinked, thereby posing a risk for HIV propagation (see Figure 5.1). About 26% and 34% of injection drug users in Karachi and Lahore, respectively, bought sex from a female sex worker, which creates a transmission pathway from injectors to other most-at-risk populations via the commercial sex network. An important indication from the survey data is that consistent condom use was almost non-existent during these commercial sex interactions. In addition, one-fifth of female sex workers had injection drug users as sex partners, and 15% of them had non-paying partners who were drug injectors.

Although a considerable proportion of sex workers could recognize condoms, knowledge about where they could be obtained was lower (see Figure 5.2). Few female sex workers could get a condom when needed, and actual condom use in all recent commercial sex activities was low (2% in Karachi and 19% in Lahore). The important issue for further advocacy was that the use of condoms was consistently higher among women who were exposed to harm reduction interventions.

As can be seen in Figure 5.3, less than one-third of respondents sought medical treatment when they had STI-related symptoms. In term of intervention planning, this signifies the need to provide education on STI symptom recognition and information about where STI care can be sought.

Another important finding is the prevalence of STI. Prevalence of syphilis was very high among *hijra* in Karachi (60%) and among male sex workers (36%) (see Figure 5.4). Prevalence of gonorrhoea was the highest among female sex workers (10% in Karachi and 12% in Lahore), as was the prevalence of chlamydia (5% in Karachi and 11% in Lahore).

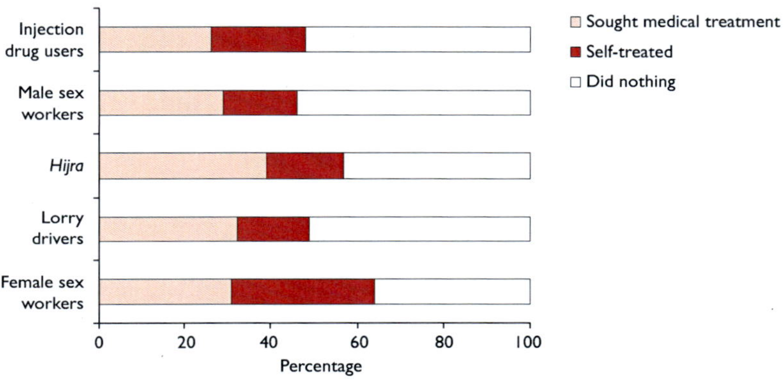

Figure 5.3 STI care–seeking behaviour, according to risk group

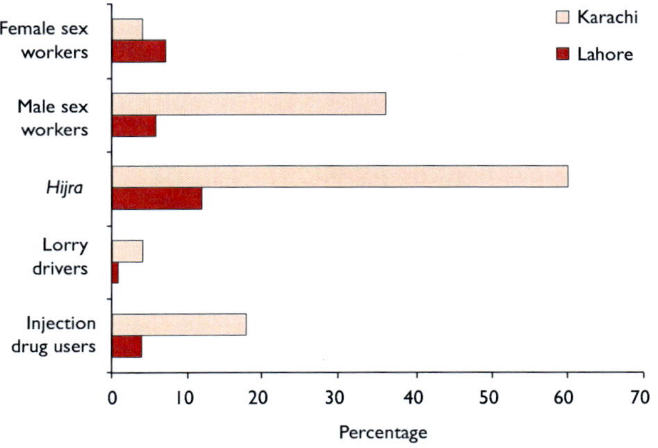

Figure 5.4 Prevalence of syphilis among most-at-risk populations

Rectal gonorrhoea was found among 29.4% of *hijra* and 17.5% of male sex workers in Karachi. What significance do these findings have for planning STI services for these most-at-risk populations? First, the high prevalence of active syphilis in *hijra* and male sex workers means that current levels of risky sexual behaviour are high, and this requires provision of screening and treatment. Second, use of condoms and provision of free condoms and lubricants for anal sex should be more actively advocated. Third, there is a clear need to expand STI services to these most-at-risk populations.

Due to the high prevalence of HIV among injection drug users, it was concluded that services prioritizing them should include easy access to sterile needles and syringes, promotion of safe sex, VCT and HIV harm reduction programmes, including in prisons.

5.6

Data dissemination

Data that have been collected, collated, analysed and interpreted are of limited use if not disseminated and acted on (Box 5.1). The aim of surveillance data dissemination is to present results of particular surveillance activities, or the key annual outcomes from the surveillance system, to those who use the data [13]. For this reason data dissemination constitutes an important component of surveillance.

Key components of the communication cycle to disseminate data include[1]:

- determining communication objectives
- establishing the message
- identifying the audience
- selecting the channel
- creating communication tools
- evaluating the impact.

After surveillance data have been analysed and interpreted, a stakeholders meeting or a workshop should be organized with key partners who work on HIV, including relevant ministries, donors, nongovernmental organizations that implement harm reduction programmes and members and representatives of the populations affected by HIV. Dissemination workshops must include the priority populations to inform them of what is happening with respect to HIV in their communities. These workshops can also raise their interest in participation and collaboration in subsequent surveillance surveys. The full surveillance report or briefing reports are presented during such dissemination workshops. The outline and scope of such reports will depend on the audience. Important participants at such dissemination workshops are providers who collect data and constitute the surveillance front line since such feedback of results and acknowledgement of their efforts will enhance their willingness to participate in sentinel surveillance activities and improve the sustainability of the system.

> **Box 5.1 What are the benefits of dissemination?**
>
> - Motivates individuals or organizations to continue to be part of the surveillance activities
> - Motivates high quality data collection
> - Broadens scope of the surveillance system
> - Facilitates use of surveillance information for advocacy and evidence-based programme planning

---

[1] From *Guidelines for conducting HIV sentinel serosurveys among pregnant women and other groups*. Geneva, UNAIDS/WHO, 2003.

The methods and results of each surveillance survey should be described in a report. In addition, annual surveillance reports should be published by the national surveillance agency and disseminated to those who need to have information on the epidemiology of HIV infection in the country. The participants of surveillance data dissemination workshop can include, but should not be limited to:

- members and representatives of the priority populations
- relevant ministries: health, education, development, sex, youth, etc.
- international and nongovernmental organizations concerned with HIV surveillance
- organizations that provide services to the priority groups
- staff that participate in surveillance
- academic institutions as key partners in implementation and education.

The visual presentation of data in graphs and figures helps to quickly and clearly convey the message. The key information to communicate in reports and during data dissemination workshop includes:

- key findings from the surveillance survey (or routine reporting)
- prevalence levels of HIV and STI
- key behaviour that drives these epidemics
- links among most-at-risk populations, between most-at-risk populations and to bridging populations
- current coverage with interventions in risk groups: access to and use of condoms, access to and use of VCT, ability to get sterile injecting equipment when needed, access to HIV- and STI-related education
- recommendations for actions in terms of further development of prevention, treatment and care
- recommendations for actions in terms of surveillance system improvement.

Data can be made available in a variety of formats to facilitate their use and application, and the presentation and the means of communication will depend on the target audience. Multiple methods now exist, and surveillance experts should maximize the use of available technologies for the greatest effect. Surveillance information can be disseminated by various communication channels including:

- annual surveillance reports with the key results from all surveillance activities conducted and the relevance of findings for prevention and control
- reports from specific surveillance surveys with key findings from the groups covered
- epidemiological bulletins and newsletters
- scientific journals and conferences
- electronic mail to surveillance staff at regional and local levels
- web pages of the surveillance institutions (it may involve password-protected access to some information)
- briefing reports for policy-makers and programme managers
- press releases—it is important that they concisely and in a non-stigmatizing manner explain the main findings and the prevention messages.

Reports from surveillance surveys should include the following sections:

- executive summary
- rationale for the survey
- aim and objectives
- methods, including
  - process of pre-surveillance assessment and fieldwork: number of experts and key informants interviewed, results of interviews, lists of sites reported by informants and experts, results of mapping, estimated number of people at venues, principles of cluster selection, recruitment of individuals
  - sample size (expected and achieved sample size)
  - biological tests performed
- results of the data analysis with a list of key indicators; proportion of non-respondents
- problems encountered during the fieldwork and limitations of the survey (participation and refusal rates, safety problems, problems with transportation of specimens, etc.)
- recommendations for HIV prevention and care programmes based on the data
- appendixes with data collection instruments, further details of methods, additional data tables.

Releasing certain information may cause harm, especially to vulnerable groups. Investigators should carefully assess what published information may cause harm to vulnerable groups. For example, the specific venues for recruitment should not be revealed, nor should data be presented in a manner that may reveal the identities of persons or appear to identify persons. Agencies conducting surveillance activities that may potentially harm those at risk have the obligation to use the data to maximize benefits to the same populations. At the same time, interpretation of data has to be consistent with scientific integrity [14].

Additional challenges that surveillance data dissemination may bring include:

- lowering the priority given to HIV and STI
- overloading the public and health professionals with information
- misinterpretation of data by the press and public
- further stigmatization of affected communities.

5.7

Evaluation of HIV surveillance systems

Why do we evaluate?

The aim of the evaluation of an HIV surveillance system is to ensure that the system is monitoring effectively the course of the HIV epidemic and contributing to development of HIV prevention, care and treatment activities. Evaluation assesses the utility of the system for decision-making, treatment, care and prevention, and further HIV research. Evaluation of a surveillance system is a learning tool and forms a basis for improving the existing system. Evaluation can be internal, which is usually carried out annually, or external, which is carried out by experts outside of the surveillance institutions and can be undertaken every few years. The methods and results of the evaluation of a surveillance system need to be defined in the surveillance workplan, and the results of the evaluation should be written into the annual surveillance reports.

This section is based on the CDC publication *Updated guidelines for evaluating public health surveillance systems* [15], available at http://www.cdc.gov/mmwr/preview/mmwrhtml/rr5013a1.htm.

A general framework for evaluating a public health surveillance system consists of the following steps:

- engage stakeholders
- identify and clarify objectives
- describe the system
- assess system performance
- draw conclusions and make recommendations
- communicate the evaluation.

Engage stakeholders

Stakeholder contribution helps ensure inclusion of all issues vital to the surveillance system evaluation. Stakeholders can be representatives from the national institution responsible for HIV surveillance, local/regional surveillance institutions, those who collect or provide data (physicians, academic institutions, nongovernmental organizations), staff from the national HIV reference laboratory, researchers involved in population-based HIV surveys and international and funding agencies. They provide inputs to the needs to upgrade any aspects of the system and more effectively use data for HIV prevention, control and treatment.

Identify and clarify objectives

At the beginning of the evaluation, the main aims of evaluation need to be defined. These may include assessing the performance of the system; finding out whether the system covers all groups most at risk for HIV acquisition and transmission; revising the types of data collection sources and sampling methods according to the changing characteristics of the HIV epidemic; or assessing whether the current surveillance system is providing sufficient information on the outcome and impact indicators for evaluation of the national AIDS programme.

Describe the surveillance system

When describing the HIV surveillance system, it is useful to find out whether there is a strategic plan for HIV surveillance which defines the functions, roles and responsibilities of those who participate in surveillance, its aims and objectives, and whether it is a part of the national AIDS programme. In addition, there should also be a workplan that details activities along with associated timelines and budgets. The HIV surveillance system should be guided and planned by a surveillance coordinating committee.

Other issues that need to be addressed when describing the system are:

- the public health importance of the health-related event under surveillance (in this case, HIV and related behaviour)
- the purpose and operation of the system
- the resources used to operate the system
- the existence and quality of protocols for each surveillance survey.

General parameters for measuring the importance of a health-related event under surveillance include several components:

- indexes of frequency (the total number of cases and/or deaths; incidence rates; prevalence; mortality rates) and summary measures of population health status (such as quality-adjusted life years)
- indexes of severity (case–fatality ratio, hospitalization rates, disability rates)
- inequities associated with the health-related event
- economic costs associated with the health-related event
- preventability
- public interest and perception.

When describing the purpose and operation of the public health surveillance system, we need to address the following issues:

- the objectives of the system
- the planned uses of data from the system
- what the health-related events under HIV surveillance are, including the case definitions used for HIV and AIDS
- who has the legal obligation for data collection and reporting

- which institutions are responsible for the surveillance system management (draw a flow chart of the system)
- the level of integration with other systems (with TB surveillance, and integration of HIV and STI surveillance)
- the components of the system such as:
  - o the population groups under surveillance
  - o the type of data collected and design of the surveillance surveys
  - o the reporting sources for routine HIV case reporting
  - o the procedures for data management in terms of transfer, entry, editing, storage and backup
  - o the analysis and dissemination plans for the system's data
  - o the policies and procedures in place to ensure patient privacy, data confidentiality and system security.

The resources used to run the system also need to be described. They include operational funding, personnel that work on data collection and analysis and those that manage and coordinate the system, as well as other resources such as travel, training, equipment and laboratory support.

Describe the system performance

An assessment of how the system is performing is the key element of the evaluation. It consists of a description of the following attributes of the system:

- simplicity
- flexibility
- data quality
- acceptability
- sensitivity
- positive predictive value
- representativeness
- timeliness
- stability.

Simplicity refers to the structure and ease of operations, which should be clearly explained to all who participate in surveillance. The notion that surveillance systems should be simple is not easy to apply to HIV surveillance systems as they have become complex, with many sources of information.

Flexibility refers to the ability of the system to adapt to changing needs with little additional time and funding.

Data quality relates primarily to the completeness and validity of the data. One of the ways to assess data quality is to examine the percentage of "unknown" and "missing responses" in surveillance data forms. Many issues influence data quality, such as the clarity of surveillance data forms and questionnaires, the representativeness of survey data, the quality of supervision and the validity of laboratory tests. In sentinel surveillance, data should be analysed by site, which allows for the identification of sites that do not report consistently and any other errors.

Acceptability reflects the willingness of persons and organizations to participate in the surveillance system. Acceptability is measured by estimating the number of agencies or individual practitioners who participate in surveillance out of all those who were asked to participate, the completeness of data collection forms and timeliness of reporting. Acceptability also depends on how key stakeholders perceive the public health importance of HIV, the extent to which the system acknowledges their contribution, feedback to data providers, responsiveness of the system to comments and time taken by data collection.

Sensitivity can be described as the ability of the surveillance system to detect cases and outbreaks and changes in HIV-related behaviour and HIV prevalence over time. The sensitivity will be influenced by the extent to which people can be tested and the accessibility of testing for those most at risk, the extent of reporting to surveillance institutions, and the quality of the implementation of HIV surveys that measure prevalence. To estimate sensitivity, it is necessary to compare different data sources, such as prevalence surveys and routine reporting and to get estimates on the extent of (under)reporting in the passive case reporting system. Also, the number of HIV cases diagnosed at laboratories can be compared to those reported to the surveillance institution by physicians.

Positive predictive value (PPV) is the proportion of reported cases that actually have the infection or disease of interest. PPV depends on the specificity of the test or case definition and the prevalence of infection in the population.

Representativeness is the extent to which surveillance data can be generalized to the population they represent. The highest generalizability can be achieved by conducting studies that are based on probability sampling methods. Multiple sources of surveillance data enable triangulation—the exploration of the extent to which different surveillance data sources are comparable and can be used to validate one another. It is also necessary to elucidate the role of private providers in HIV testing, care and treatment, and their contribution to reporting.

Timeliness is the speed between different actions in public health surveillance. In case reporting, it is the time between case detection and the reporting of that event to public health authorities. Timeliness can also be described as the time required to detect trends and outbreaks, and, if possible, the effectiveness of control measures. In describing timeliness, it is also necessary to find out how often bio-behavioural prevalence surveys are conducted, and whether this frequency meets the needs of monitoring trends. The frequency of repetition of surveillance surveys depends on the baseline findings, the expected rate of change, and the availability of financial resources. In general, results that we get from baseline surveys should allow us to set surveillance priorities for the future. Institution-based surveillance often runs annually or every other year, while community-based studies are repeated every several years.

Stability refers to the ability of the system to work properly and without failure. It can be assessed as the number of times that the electronic system breaks down, staff turnover, the amount of time needed to manage data (including data transfer, entry and editing), and time needed to analyse and report the data.

Conclusions and recommendations

The report on the evaluation should outline the main findings including a description of the system and its attributes and the system's performance. It is important to suggest what steps are necessary to improve the system and to be better able to monitor the epidemic more effectively, and how this can be achieved. It should also outline the cost of these new activities and what benefits improvements in the system would bring to understanding HIV transmission and the development of HIV prevention and control. The recommendations for the system improvement should also balance the increase in the quality of the system's performance with costs.

Communication

The result of the evaluation should be communicated to the surveillance team and to the key stakeholders, such as the national AIDS programme, the ministry of health and the key agencies and institutions that contribute to data collection. It aims to inform the key stakeholders about the outcomes of the evaluation, primarily the overall performance of the HIV surveillance system and what steps and actions are necessary for its improvement.

References

1   Štulhofer A, Ajduković D, Božičević I, Kufrin K. *HIV/AIDS and youth in Croatia. The study of sexual behaviour, practices and attitudes* [in Croatian]. Final report. Zagreb, Ministry of Health, 2006.

2   Walker N, Stover J, Stanecki K, Zaniewski AE, Grassly NC, Garcia-Calleja JM, Ghys PD. The workbook approach to making estimates and projecting future scenarios of HIV/AIDS in countries with low level and concentrated epidemics. *Sexually transmitted infections*, 2004, 80 (suppl 1):i10–i13.

3   Ghys PD, Brown T, Grassly NC, Garnett G, Stanecki KA, Stover J, Walker N. The UNAIDS Estimation and Projection Package: a software package to estimate and project national HIV epidemics. *Sexually transmitted infections*, 2004, 80(suppl 1): i5–i9.

4   *Development of the software packages, EPP v2 and Spectrum, and measuring and tracking the epidemic in countries where HIV is concentrated among populations at high risk of HIV.* Report of a meeting of the UNAIDS Reference Group for Estimates, Modelling and Projections held in Sintra, Portugal, 8–10 December 2004.

5   RDS Analysis Tool v5.6. User manual. New York, RDS Incorporated, 2006. Available at http://www.respondentdrivensampling.org/.

6   Jordan-Harder B, Maboko L, Mmbando D, Riedner G, Nagele E, Harder J, Kuchen V, Kilian A, Korte R, Sonnenburg FV. Thirteen year HIV-1 sentinel surveillance and indicators for behavioural change suggest impact of programme activities in south-west Tanzania. *AIDS*, 2004, 18 (2):287–94.

7   Zaba B, Slaymaker E, Urassa M, Boerma JT. The role of behavioral data in HIV surveillance. *AIDS*, 2005, 19(suppl 2):S39–S52.

8   *Case study. Country-enhanced monitoring & evaluation for antiretroviral therapy scale-up: analysis and use of strategic information in Botswana.* San Francisco, World Health Organization, Institute for Global Health, 2006. Available at http://www.igh.org/news/Botswana2006.pdf.

9   Thacker SB, Berkelman RL, Stroup DF. The science of public health surveillance. *Journal of public health policy*, 1989, 10(2):187–203.

10   Garcia-Calleja JM, Gouws E, Ghys PD. National population based HIV prevalence surveys in sub-Saharan Africa: results and implications for HIV and AIDS estimates. *Sexually transmitted infections*, 2006, 82(suppl 3):iii64–iii70.

11 Pisani EO, Garnett GP, Brown T, Stover J, Grassly NC, Hankins C, et al. Back to basics in HIV prevention: focus on exposure. *British medical journal*, 2003, 326:1384–7.

12 *International ethical guidelines for biomedical research involving human subjects.* Geneva, Council for International Organizations of Medical Sciences, 2002.

13 Mandel JS, Rutherford GW. AIDS prevention research in low and middle-income countries: increasing the dissemination of study results in the scientific literature. *AIDS and behavior*, 2006, 10:S1–S4.

14 *International guidelines for ethical review of epidemiological studies.* Geneva, Council for International Organizations of Medical Sciences, 1991.

15 Updated guidelines for evaluating public health surveillance systems. Recommendations from the Guidelines Working Group. *Morbidity and mortality weekly report*, 2001, 50(RR13):1–35. Available at http://www.cdc.gov/mmwr/preview/mmwrhtml/rr5013a1.htm.